PRAISE FOR *FED UP!*

"*Fed Up!* is an affirming and intelligent gift to women and men. Dr. Oliver-Pyatt has done what makes for magical teaching, that is to deliver a message that is informed by both heart and intellect."

—Barbara Kohlenberg, Ph.D, Clinical
Psychologist, V.A. Sierra Nevada Health
Network

"In a compelling and professional voice, Dr. Oliver-Pyatt provides a deeper understanding of what lies at the heart of overeating, and disordered eating, offering hope for those who are ready for an innovative approach toward life-long physical and mental health and well-being."

—Anita M. Sacks, C.S.W., L.C.S.W., A.C.S.W.,
Clinical Instructor of Psychiatry, New York
University School of Medicine, Member,
Institute for Psychoanalytic Training and
Research, New York City

"*Fed Up!* is a engaging book that is both personally and professionally useful. Firmly grounded in science, *Fed Up!* provides an action plan that will put the reader on the road to better physical and mental health. Health care professionals will find *Fed Up!* a great help in working with individuals who are struggling with weight control and self-image problems."

—John N. Chappel, M.D., Professor Emeritus
of Psychiatry, University of Nevada
School of Medicine

"*Fed Up!* combines a very honest exploration of Dr. Oliver-Pyatt's personal struggles with food and weight with her expertise as a physician. The result is an accessible step-wise program that restores a natural relationship between you, your body, and food."

—Kristin Beizai, M.D., Assistant Professor of
Psychiatry, University of Tennesse

"In *Fed Up!*, Dr. Oliver-Pyatt has composed a masterful book. It is subtitled *The Breakthrough Ten-Step, No-Diet Fitness Plan*, but it is so much more than any conventional "how-to" guide. Dr. Oliver-Pyatt manages to place the pursuit of a healthy body weight in the context of the larger frame of psychological health. Anyone struggling with unhappiness about their body, and anyone living with someone who is desperately buying into the hopeless diet frenzy, ought to get their hands on this book."

—Ole J. Thienhaus, M.D., M.B.A., Professor
of Psychiatry, Chairman, Department of
Psychiatry, University of Nevada, School of
Medicine, Adjunct Professor of Psychology

"*Fed Up!* is a revolutionary book that clearly outlines the keys to a relaxed relationship with food, a diet-free life, and long-term fitness. If you're tired of useless diets and weight-loss schemes, this comprehensive ten-step plan offers an answer worth seeking."

—Brenda Erickson, M.D., Board Certified
Psychiatrist and Eating Disorder Specialist

Fed Up!

Fed Up!

The Breakthrough Ten-Step, No-Diet Fitness Plan

WENDY OLIVER-PYATT, M.D.

Contemporary Books

Chicago   New York   San Francisco   Lisbon   London   Madrid   Mexico City
Milan   New Delhi   San Juan   Seoul   Singapore   Sydney   Toronto

Library of Congress Cataloging-in-Publication Data

Oliver-Pyatt, Wendy.
　　Fed Up! : the breakthrough ten-step, no-diet fitness plan / Wendy Oliver-
　Pyatt.
　　　　p.　cm.
　　ISBN 0-07-138331-X
　　1. Weight loss.　　2. Physical fitness.　　I. Title.

RM222.2.O42　　2003
613.7—dc21　　　　　　　　　　　　　　　　　　　2002020759

Contemporary Books

A Division of The **McGraw-Hill** *Companies*

1 2 3 4 5 6 7 8 9 0　AGM/AGM　1 0 9 8 7 6 5 4 3 2

ISBN 0-07-138331-X

McGraw-Hill books are available at special quantity discounts to use as premiums and
sales promotions, or for use in corporate training programs. For more information,
please write to the Director of Special Sales, Professional Publishing, McGraw-Hill,
Two Penn Plaza, New York, NY 10121-2298. Or contact your local bookstore.

Consult a physician before beginning this or any other weight-loss or fitness
plan. Certain medical conditions may require modification of the advice
provided in this book.

This book is printed on acid-free paper.

For Mikaela and Jada

Contents

PREFACE

I BEGIN THIS book by explaining how our culture programs us to diet, and why diets don't work. I encourage you to read those chapters carefully, because awareness is the first step toward changing your life for the better.

But this book isn't merely a thesis on why we diet and why diets fail. In Parts II through IV, I'll show you how to transform your new awareness into positive actions that can free you from weight problems forever.

Many of you try diet after diet with no success, while others have given up on the idea of ever reaching your ideal body weight. No matter what form your struggle with weight takes, the Ten-Step No-Diet Fitness Plan that follows will enable you to lose excess pounds permanently and to have a relaxed relationship with food.

This is my wish for you.
Dr. Wendy Oliver-Pyatt

ACKNOWLEDGMENTS

FEW BOOKS ARE written in isolation, and *Fed Up!* has benefited enormously from the wise advice and creative contributions of many friends.

I would like to start by thanking Dr. David Salvage for encouraging me to believe that this book was within my reach. His energy, inspiration, and vision were invaluable when I began this book. Dr. Salvage is a deep-thinking and compassionate psychiatrist, and his friendship and collegiality are greatly appreciated.

Heidi von Gnechten-Wright was extremely helpful in reading *Fed Up!* and editing the entire manuscript. Heidi's contribution and friendship are a most generous gift.

I would also like to thank my dear friend Vicki Kroviak for our eighteen-year friendship, her never-ending support, and her insightful contributions to this book. In addition, I greatly appreciate the perspective of her husband, Steve Grieder, whose comments greatly improved *Fed Up!*

I am also grateful to Alison Blake, for helping me put into words the stories and concepts I wished to share.

My heartfelt thanks go out to my agent, Margot Maley Hutchison, and my editor, Betsy Lancefield Lane. Because Margot and Betsy believed in my ideas, and in me, *Fed Up!* exists as a book and not just an idea in my mind. Also, I thank Nancy Hall, my project editor, for transforming the manuscript into this book and for making it such a smooth, friendly, and fun process.

I thank Bill, Diana, Shirley, Julie, Kathy, Melissa M., Melissa W., Tracy, Leah, Lisa, Charlene, David, Sandy, and all of the people who have been there for me, for friendship and support.

My gratitude also goes to the New York University Department of Psychiatry and all of its fantastically rich teaching sites including Bellevue Hospital, Lenox Hill Hospital, and Manhattan Psychiatric Institute for providing me with a most interesting and rewarding training program in psychiatry and for exposing me to those conditions that allowed my fullest growth during a critical time in my life. I thank the many colleagues and supervisors who supported me and offered their insights, expertise, and wisdom. I thank Anita Sacks, A.C.S.W., L.C.S.W.; Jim Halper, M.D.; and Shelley Orgel, M.D., all tremendous supervisors who contributed to my development and made a lasting impression on me.

I give thanks especially to all of my patients, who are my unsurpassed teachers, and who challenge me to be and do my best; in doing so, they continuously contribute to my growth.

Thanks also go to my brothers, Mark and Glen Oliver. Their presence in my life is a source of comfort and strength. I thank my father, Michael Oliver, for always thinking big.

A special note of love and appreciation goes to the memory of my mother, Betty.

My two daughters, Mikaela and Jada, have been the greatest gift in my life. I give thanks for their health, their warm spirit, and the opportunity to watch them grow.

Finally, I thank my husband, Michael Pyatt. His gentle manner, companionship, and wisdom are admired and appreciated each day of my life. He has always given his fullest support to my personal and professional development. The happiness and stability that his presence brings to my life have enabled me to put forth the creative energy necessary to turn my memories of years of dieting and self-denial into a book that I hope will allow others to achieve lifelong mental and physical fitness without dieting.

INTRODUCTION

IF YOU'VE TRIED Sugar Busters, Weight Watchers, Body for Life, the Atkins diet, and Jenny Craig, and still can't achieve permanent weight loss, now is the time for a new approach—an approach that goes beyond the superficial hype of the diet books pumped out year after year by the diet industry. If you're ready for a change, and for a healthy and attractive body, it's time to get **Fed Up.**

Why? Because dieting isn't making you lose weight—it's making you gain it. In this book, I'll tell you exactly how to reverse the relentless spiral and achieve the beautiful body you deserve. (Yes, you can lose those excess pounds—for good!) But first you need to get mad about what the diet industry is doing to you and to millions of other Americans who buy into its myths.

Why Get Fed Up?

Let's admit it: we all know that dieting doesn't work. We either gain the weight back every time or live in a nonstop war with food and our bodies. Each diet is harder and harder, and each time we "rebound," we add more pounds than we lost and replace muscle with fat.

But dieting does more than hurt our bodies. It hurts our souls, and each failed diet makes the wound deeper.

How does dieting damage us?

When our self-esteem revolves around our weight and our perception of our bodies as inadequate, we cannot take our emotional state seriously.

When we are more preoccupied with counting every calorie than we are about our needs, we are not connected with our inner life.

When we buy clothes that are the wrong size, thinking that we will fit into them after we diet, we are not living in the present and we are lying to ourselves.

When we eat to feel better, less depressed, and less anxious or to control our anger or numb ourselves, we are hurting ourselves.

When we begin a diet to look good for a holiday or a party, we are playing a dangerous game with our physical and mental health.

When we diet to become thinner and more lovable, we are in fact setting ourselves up for failure.

When we compare ourselves with women or men in magazines displaying unrealistic beauty ideals and believe we are deficient, we are treating ourselves with disrespect.

When our lives and emotions focus more on concern about our body shape and the food we eat than on loving ourselves, respecting ourselves, and celebrating ourselves, we are cheating ourselves and those who love us.

In our attempts to attain happiness by dieting our way to an ideal body, we move farther and farther away from happiness—and, ironically, farther away from our goal of looking attractive, feeling healthy, and achieving long-term weight loss.

Who Are We?

We are a diverse group. Some of us are married; others are divorced, in relationships, or single. Some of us come from highly functional families; some don't. We are doctors, artists, homemakers, attorneys, realtors, and athletes. We are everywhere, in every size and age and color. Most of us are women, but more and more men are joining our ranks. And many of us share some or all of these feelings:

- We are deeply disturbed by and unhappy with our bodies. Many of us allow this unhappiness to consume a vast amount of our energy. Others of us disconnect from the emotional pain that weight issues cause us and refuse to take our bodies or our minds seriously.

- We struggle with our self-esteem and find that it revolves around our body size and weight.
- We desire perfection in our bodies and feel that we are failures if we are unable to achieve it.
- We believe that a thin body holds the key to happiness.
- We may set extraordinarily high standards for ourselves but sometimes don't expect enough from others.
- We have difficulty accepting the validity of our feelings and needs.
- We tend to be secretive about our eating and about the degree to which we are unhappy because of our body size.
- We use food to dampen our feelings yet feel worse as a result.

There are millions of us. We're people who sit in restaurants ordering salads, envying the people eating steaks at the next table. We're people who graze on food to cope with anxiety and then feel weak and ashamed. We're people who've abandoned the idea of ever achieving long-term weight loss, feeling that it's beyond our reach. We're people who settle for less-than-healthy relationships, believing that we don't deserve better because we're not svelte enough. We're highly competent, successful women and men who refuse to go swimming in public because we're ashamed of our bodies. And we're targets for the multibillion-dollar weight-loss industry, which entices us each week with new diets, weight-loss creams, expensive exercise equipment, and body wraps.

Many of us learn early on that these magic "cures" for being overweight are worthless, and we give up on the idea that we will ever be a healthy or normal weight. Consigned to live in bodies we hate, we lead lives suffused with dissatisfaction and self-loathing.

For many others of us, eating preoccupations become a way of life. We wake up thinking about what we ate the day before. We weigh ourselves before we eat breakfast. We judge whether a day is good or bad based not on what we learned, enjoyed, or accomplished but on whether we've gained or lost a pound. We worry about gaining weight and about our bellies and our breasts hanging. We relish the "rush" of getting on the scale and seeing the numbers drop and feel deep despair when we break down and go off our rigid regimens and gain the pounds back. We binge or emotionally graze, filling ourselves with food while our emptiness remains profound and nameless. We diet because we are afraid that we want more than what is good for us and because we fear our hunger is bottomless.

And we always fail. Even if we succeed in controlling our weight temporarily, our diets teach us that we cannot trust our instincts or ourselves. We are unable to have a relaxed relationship with food, and some of us find it difficult to have healthy relationships with other people—our spouses, lovers, parents, and children—because our issues with food and our bodies take central importance in our lives. There is no part of our psychic and physical lives that food does not impact.

For some of us, dieting becomes a disease or even a death sentence. We become anorexics and bulimics, seeking even more dangerous goals of thinness at any cost. Others—the "typical" dieters among us—go through life quietly crippled by our food preoccupations. And still others of us say "Enough" and give up, convinced that we will always want too much and believing that we can never achieve a healthy body weight and size.

To other people, our ordeal is invisible. But it rules our lives. We pick up magazines, not to read the articles but to try yet another diet plan. We fantasize about a world where food has no calories and our bodies are always perfect. We feel sick and weak when we eat "bad" foods and deprived and weary when we force ourselves to avoid them. Every piece of fattening food becomes an emotional crisis, from a piece of wedding cake at a reception to a box of leftover pizza in the refrigerator. We put food down the disposal or throw it in the trash to avoid eating it. Some of us throw up the food we do eat or take laxatives to remove it from our bodies. Others of us seek emotional comfort and pleasure from food, while suffering intense shame and the disapproval of a culture that labels us as weak-willed for being overweight. To all of us, no matter what form our problems take, the idea of food as natural, fun, or necessary is alien.

I say "we" and "us," because this is my story, too. Like the women and men this book is about, I spent years of my life trapped in the prison of *weight cycling*—the medical term for an agonizing merry-go-round of losing weight, gaining weight, starving, and bingeing. I know what it's like to live on salad and low-fat dressing for weeks, only to gorge on a carton of ice cream. I understand how it feels to struggle for weeks to lose five pounds and then gain it back within days. I know the shame, pain, and hopelessness of failed dieting. I know how it feels to envy other women who eat without fear and those who have seemingly perfect bodies.

It took me years to realize that despite my deep desire for thinness, the approach I was using—the constant diets, the constant deprivation, the inevitable bingeing—did not and could not work. Instead, it caused me massive amounts of pain and guilt and rendered me incapable of enjoying my life. I wanted out—and, through a long process of self-discovery, I found the way.

Today I live in a house full of ice cream, Popsicles, leftover macaroni and cheese, and boxes of Chinese takeout. I eat them whenever I'm hungry. I never feel deprived. And I don't worry about gaining weight, because I'm in control of my eating, and my life, again.

My experience has led me, as a psychiatrist, to take special interest in the issues of food preoccupations and dieting and to develop an effective plan to help other women (and a growing number of men) escape from a lifetime of unhappiness about their bodies. When these women and men grow to understand the cultural, psychological, and biological reasons why they diet, why their diets don't work, and why it's a mistake to believe that weight loss is unattainable, they begin the process of transformation to self-acceptance and self-control. They learn how to eat without fear and to keep their bodies healthy and attractive—permanently.

As you read this book, you may fear trying something new. But you must ask yourself, what do you have to lose? Do you want to continue to live in the cage in which endless dieting or compulsive overeating traps you—or do you long to leave that cage and live a life in which you are happy with yourself and your body, you look and feel great, and food is a simple pleasure and not a torment?

If you've picked up this book, I believe you're ready to take the first step toward freedom and real fitness. I hope you will let me—as a fellow traveler and a guide who once walked the same path—offer you the road map that can release you, once and for all, from weight and food preoccupations and give you the beautiful body that's within your reach.

What will you gain? A sexy, attractive, healthy body. A healthy mind. The energy and freedom to do what you want with your life. A release from the guilt, low self-esteem, and self-flagellation that compulsive dieting often causes. The realization that you can be fit without maintaining a constant "diet mentality." And the knowledge that you are in control—and you will never need to fear being fat again.

Part I

Get Fed Up!

*Why You Need to **Stop** Dieting
to **Start** Losing Weight*

WHILE WE'RE SPENDING more money, time, and energy than ever on weight-loss products and plans, we have the highest rate of obesity of any society in history. The clear message: what we're doing isn't working. Here's why.

My Journey

WHO AM I to tell you that you can lose weight, permanently and healthily, without dieting?

It's a good question. To begin with, I'm a medical doctor—but doctors have betrayed you before. They've given you photocopied diet lists and pep talks and told you, "All you need is willpower," and when their diets failed, they've wounded you with their condescension and disapproval. So even though weight loss is one of my specialties, I don't expect you to believe me simply because of the *M.D.* after my name.

But I'm an expert on weight loss for another reason: I sacrificed more than a decade of my life to dieting and found out the hard way that diets don't work. I tried low-cal and low-carb diets, fasting, salad-only diets, the TWA stewardess diet—you name it. Eventually I became so trapped by dieting that I put my mental and physical health at risk—yet I still didn't lose weight.

My story has a happy ending, however. My medical training, combined with my personal experiences, finally convinced me that to lose weight I had to do something counterintuitive: *I had to stop dieting.* Through a process of trial and error, I discovered a way out of the prison of dieting and into a new world. In this world I eat what I want and I maintain my desired weight easily. I never starve or sacrifice, I don't spend hours in the gym trying to sweat off calories, and I never—never—worry about losing control when I'm around food.

Better yet, I've discovered that the steps that freed me from dieting work for others as well. They work for my friends. They work for my patients. And they will work for you. You *can* achieve long-term weight loss, if you follow my Ten-Step No-Diet Fitness Plan diligently.

How did I discover the path from diet preoccupation to diet-free fitness and health? It was a long road and sometimes a dangerous one.

> *Nancy and I stood in line at the movie theater's concession counter. We both ordered popcorn—"No butter, please"—and waited to pay. As we watched, the concession clerk picked up a tub of popcorn and squirted butter into it. Simultaneously, nearly throwing ourselves over the counter, we said, "No butter!" Irritated, the clerk said, "This isn't yours."*
>
> *We'd panicked because it was unacceptable, in our world, to eat butter. Butter meant fat. And if we were fat, we'd be pathetic and alone the rest of our lives.*

I was nineteen and a premed student at the University of Denver. I had a grade point average of nearly 4.0, and my future seemed limitless. I dated interesting men, and I had close female friends. From the outside, my life probably looked perfect. Other women may have even envied me. It was ironic, because they had no way of knowing that I desperately envied *them*.

I watched them at football games, eating hot dogs and nachos. I saw them arguing politics over pizza, buying candy bars at the Student Center, or making late-night runs to McDonald's or the International House of Pancakes. I couldn't do any of these things, because all of them involved food—and food was the enemy.

Looking back, I can remember that I first started to worry about food, weight, and my body when I reached puberty. Two incidents stand out in my mind, marking the beginning of my knowledge that my body was "wrong"— too big, too feminine, too round.

When I was in sixth grade, I spent a night at my ballet teacher's house and realized the next morning that I had no clean clothes for school. "Don't worry," my teacher said and asked her daughter, who was about my age, to lend me a pair of jeans. Until that point I'd never really compared other girls' bodies to my own. But as I tried to squeeze into Donna's petite jeans—first standing up, then lying down—I realized how tiny her body was compared to mine. I could just barely squeeze my hips into the jeans, but no amount of sucking, squeezing, or squirming would allow me to zip them up. Instead of seeing my developing body as evidence of my femininity, I suddenly saw it as something grotesquely fat and misshapen.

A year or so later, a second incident helped to convince me that my fears about my weight must be valid. I was thirteen years old and trying out for cheerleader at my junior high school. I asked my older brother, whose approval I craved, what he thought of my figure.

His reply stunned me: "You look a little sloppy."

Moreover, he said, I had large thighs. At 5'7" and 130 pounds, I suddenly was labeled, by myself and by others I respected, as unacceptably fat.

I started my first diet then, talking my mother into paying to send me to a weight-loss center—an act she never questioned, reinforcing my belief that my body was too big. Every week the program staff weighed me, celebrating with me when I reached 125. The weight kept coming back, however, and eventually I discovered diet pills. For the next several years I "watched my weight," a cheerful euphemism for my unsuccessful struggle to tame my exuberantly female form into model thinness.

At the beginning, dieting was almost fun, like a frustrating but challenging game. I remember going on the TWA stewardess diet with my friend Tara, a four-day diet that limited us to peculiar food combinations such as cauliflower and lamb chops on day two. (Hamburger patties and apples on day three were a thrill.) Tara kissed me out of sheer joy after she weighed herself on day five and discovered that she had, in fact, lost ten pounds. But she gained the weight back in two weeks, and so did I.

I tried diet after diet, and with each failure dieting became less a challenge and more a battle. In time dieting stopped being something I could laugh about—"No cake for me, or I'll be fat as a cow tomorrow!"—and became the focus of my life. The change was so gradual, so subtle, that I had no idea that dieting and my quest for weight loss were damaging my health and my psyche.

My struggle with weight reached its climax when I became a young woman. In college, living in the dorm away from my chaotic but familiar home, I frequently became overwhelmed with a faceless, floating anxiety I couldn't name. As the months went by, food, and my need to control my intake of it, insidiously became the defining force in my life. But increasingly, when the anxiety struck, my control disappeared. I would find myself becoming detached, as though the world around me were unreal, and I would turn to food and eat shocking quantities of it.

When I binged, I was in a temporary state of altered consciousness, a euphoric daze. After years of dieting, food had evolved to represent something more far-reaching and intense than a simple physical need. It was the forbidden indulgence, providing temporary but powerful comfort during a binge but causing terrible shame and guilt afterward.

I can't pinpoint the exact time when dieting, and my pursuit of an "ideal" body size, became an obsession. It happened gradually and inexorably, as each diet left me less and less able to regulate my food intake by robbing me of my ability to sense my internal cues of satiety and well-being. At some point I stopped eating when I was hungry and ate only when my current diet "let" me. I stopped looking at food as delicious or fun or satisfying and started looking at it as "good" or "bad"—"good" foods being those that wouldn't add inches to my body and "bad" foods being the forbidden ones I craved but couldn't eat. As dieting took over my life, my initial goal of losing a few pounds by occasionally dieting mutated into a constant, never-ending burden that took the joy out of each day.

By losing enough weight, I gradually began to believe, I could achieve the perfect body and all that came with it. With a slender figure I could find the right man, the perfect relationship. Magically, I could achieve the joy I was missing in my life, because being thin was the key to happiness. Inside me, hidden, was a sleeping beauty. It was my job to excavate her from under the layers of excess flesh that rendered her invisible. Gradually it became my obsession—an obsession fed by magazine articles, television models, and diet books telling me I could be thinner, more attractive, and a new person.

But there was a darker side to that fairy tale. If dieting was the key to a perfect body and perfect happiness, then my continual failures at dieting meant that I might remain forever trapped in my body—which I increasingly envisioned as large and grotesque—and, by extension, trapped in a failed life. The prospect terrified me. Each time I failed at a diet, I had to try again —harder, better, more perfectly. And each failure made me feel more and more out of control and unacceptable.

I became more secretive and withdrawn. Only one best friend truly knew about my diets, binges, and purges, because she too was in the grip of food preoccupation. Feeling singular, separate from other women, we shared our "secret" lives—lives that revolved around food and our dissatisfaction with our bodies. We filled our days and nights with diets, binges, and more diets. We filled our shelves with books on counting calories and carbohydrates and articles on how to lose weight by eating grapefruit, drinking vinegar, or fasting. We weighed our food portions on a postage scale and measured out half-cups of applesauce and quarter-cups of rice. We threw out good food that wasn't on our diet of the week. We made mental lists of things we shouldn't eat, which we usually wound up eating, and lists of things that we were "allowed" to eat but usually wound up eating in a desperate, compulsive, and joyless manner.

Eventually I no longer knew what was normal. My life became a tedious system of strategies and games that revolved around eating, food, and my perception of my body. I obsessed constantly about my ability or inability to control my weight. Hunger and all that went with it—for hunger is a deep emotional experience—frightened me. If I ate normally, I might end up bingeing. If I binged, I would either be stuck with the fat or have to purge. And so I dieted with a sense of dramatic mission. I was dieting in an attempt to create an acceptable and lovable self, although in fact I was moving farther and farther from loving myself and being capable of giving to, or enjoying, relationships or my life. I felt as if my future depended on mastering my body, on disciplining it, making it smaller, more angular, more polished. The sensation of hunger was the antithesis of that body, and so that sensation became the enemy.

> *I remember the day I said to my roommate, Nancy, "I see no reason to have bread in this house." Looking back, it is hard to believe that something as basic and innocuous as bread could have created so much anxiety and tension in me. I was terrified of bread—because I hungered for it.*

The more I attempted to control my weight, the more out of control I became and the less I could trust myself around food. As the cycle progressed, the possibility of ever having a healthy and fit body became more and more distant. Looking back, I am reminded of Sisyphus, the mortal condemned by the Greek gods to roll a rock up a hill in the scorching afternoon every day for eternity, only to see it fall back to the bottom each evening. Like him, I was condemned to spend every day struggling to lose weight, only to find myself farther and farther away from the goal of a "perfect" body.

As dieting became more central to my life, so did self-sacrifice—not only of food, but also of other desires. "I won't buy that beautiful suit until I lose ten more pounds." "I'll get a bikini next year, after I've lost fifteen more pounds." "I'll buy that jewelry when I deserve it, when I'm done with my diet."

Inevitably I progressed to ever more dangerous stages of food preoccupation. I vomited after eating or purged my body with laxatives. I became more fragile, both physically and emotionally. I withdrew from friends whom I felt didn't and couldn't understand my problem and from the campus activities I had once enjoyed. I turned down dates. When my control broke, I binged and then felt devastated afterward. Yet it was only during these binges that I could experience a momentary glimpse of how rich the world was and how much I could really have.

Like most people suffering from body and food preoccupations, I was an expert at disguising my inner pain. I functioned well in my classes, although I was almost as anxious and perfectionistic about my grades as I was about my weight. Men continued to ask me out, but I usually said no, and they probably thought I was "playing hard to get." The truth, however, was that I often avoided social situations because I felt my body was not acceptable. I often felt alone, in spite of having several good friends—friends I couldn't let fully into my secret, shameful world, no matter how loyal they were.

After a day of bingeing, I felt massive, ponderous, and innately unworthy. I would swaddle myself in dark blue sweatpants, disappearing into the loose folds of the material and for a moment feeling less bloated and repulsive. When I wore this outfit, it was a sign to my friend David that something was wrong. "You're wearing the sweats," he'd say ominously. "What's going on?" But even though he was a close friend, he only had a vague idea of how trapped I was in my warfare on the battlefield of my body.

My preoccupation with food and weight kept me psychically encapsulated, as if a thin layer of an evanescent bubble barred me from genuine contact with the people around me. Yet I felt an unrelenting gnawing of envy in my gut as I watched other people living, falling in love, being excited, and discovering themselves. My relationships with other women whose bodies were more "perfect" left me feeling diminished and envious. I frantically desired the idealized form they seemed to maintain so effortlessly and felt powerless for wanting what remained outside my reach.

As time went on, my life centered more and more around lies, not just to other people (who never knew that I sometimes sneaked off to vomit up the pizza I'd just eaten or that I compensated for nice meals by fasting the next day) but also to myself. When I was dieting, I wasn't happy, but I rationalized that dieting was better than being fat. When I binged, I told myself I deserved a break after struggling so long and so hard. And when I purged, the voice inside me, desperate and scientific, told me that I must react to the food within, in an effort to somehow unite these two worlds, to have the whole cake and eat it too.

I told myself other lies as well. At the outset of my dieting and bingeing episodes I said, "Well, I diet, but I don't have an eating disorder, because at least I don't vomit." Later, of course, I did begin vomiting up my food and then taking laxatives to purge myself of "bad" calories. At one point, when a glimmer of awareness made me frightened at what I was doing, I stopped using the laxatives and went back to simply dieting—because diets were acceptable, weren't they? My doctor, with the best of intentions, had in fact recommended a diet to me, to my mother, and to most of the other women who visited him. What could possibly be wrong with doing what my doctor had told us all to do?

As time passed, my dieting became ever more desperate. I became intolerant of vomiting and laxatives so I turned to exercise and fasting. Sometimes I went one or two days without eating at all, in a desperate attempt to compensate for a day of bingeing or for eating forbidden foods. And each time I gave in and binged, I began all over again. I felt as though I'd lived this way forever, and I didn't believe that there would ever be a way out.

For brief moments, now and then, I saw myself honestly—and in those moments I was frightened. At one of those times I went for a screening at an eating disorders program that I'd read about in the newspaper. I remember being stunned when the doctor there told me I had bulimia nervosa and recommended hospitalization. I left his office scared and sat in my car trying to collect my thoughts. A hospital? For me? Was he crazy? It was too much, too soon, for me to even begin to accept it. (No one can give up an all-consuming obsession immediately; it requires time, planning, patience, and, above all, readiness, a fact this well-intentioned doctor didn't recognize.)

Nonetheless, my visit helped me. There was power in knowing that my problem had a name—that I wasn't alone, that millions of women nationwide were doing the same "crazy" things, feeling the same exhaustion and shame. It was a first step, but the anxiety of taking that step was almost unbearable.

After I left the doctor's office, I felt the tension stirring within me. I can clearly remember that warm summer night in Denver, with a vivid sunset of crimson and plum clouds. Students were milling on the lawns of the campus, awaiting a concert by a local jazz band. They were full of excitement; I was filled with anxiety. It wasn't long before I started eating.

I started at a Mexican restaurant about half a mile from the dorm. I ate a burrito quickly, sitting in my car. I could scarcely taste it, because the emptiness was not in my mouth or my stomach but in some nameless, deeper place. I went back for a couple of tacos, and then, instead of going home, I stopped at the 7-Eleven and picked up a pint of Häagen-Dazs and some red licorice—which I'd read was healthier than other candy because it contained whole wheat—and downed them when I returned to my dorm room.

I was vaguely soothed, and yet further wounded, as the greasy food settled in my distended stomach. Emerging from the "rush" was the letdown: again, I'd failed. I sat in my room, deeply alone, and the words scrolled in my head with the random implacability of a medieval torture instrument: Ugly. Large. Unacceptable. Imperfect. It wasn't just that I was too big, I was . . . too much. Moving without volition, as if guided by a force outside myself, I grabbed my keys and headed for the store. It was embarrassing to purchase laxatives, but it was late at night and nobody would know. What I had done to myself needed to be undone.

I drove to the store, bought the laxatives, and began the drive home. And then, out of my despair that evening, came the first glimmer of light. Perhaps it was born out of fear, out of images of hospitals, but I don't think so. In retrospect I believe I was recognizing for the first time just how inexpressibly tired I was.

As I headed home from the store, I dreaded the idea of taking the laxatives. The thought of spending another evening huddled in the bathroom while other people lived real lives—listened to jazz, studied, kissed, went to movies—suddenly exhausted me. I realized, in a moment of clarity, that the doctor was right about something: I'd gone too far.

Without hesitation I rolled down the car window and flung the laxatives as far as I could. The white pills, still coated in their plastic wrappers, slid across the asphalt as I drove on, feeling courageous, reborn. I felt like a hostage who suddenly sees that freedom is a possibility.

I wasn't done dieting yet; in fact, I dieted until I reached medical school. But I had begun to wonder. What was I doing to myself? Why wasn't it working?

I'd begun to see that it wasn't about appetite or food. It was about my body and my conflicting needs to fill it and to deny its existence. It was about the belief that other people, women in particular, had something that I didn't. It was about the shadowy, flickering newsreel of my unconscious, playing out the endless scenarios of my own inadequacy. And, as my psychiatric training revealed to me, it was about cultural programming, cognitive distortions, childhood influences, psychodynamic defenses, and biological imperatives.

Sorting out the threads that held me captive in my preoccupation with weight and dieting required more years, but they were years of dawning self-awareness. Gradually I learned to trust myself, to take the risk of giving up on diets, and to change the terms I'd imposed on myself. I learned that I could surrender my rigid eating patterns without falling apart or becoming heavier. I learned to eat naturally and normally and discovered to my astonishment that I could control my appetite and my weight without diets, compulsive exercise, laxatives, vomiting, or diet pills. I learned to experience my body as lovable and beautiful, even though I wasn't razor-thin like the magazine models I'd once emulated. And, most important, I grew to accept and genuinely like the person I was. I learned to take myself seriously in all areas of my life, which allowed me to take my own hunger and need for satiation seriously as well.

I'm sitting in my kitchen with Nancy, my roommate from college, my former dieting partner, and still a close friend. We're listening to classical music, letting the harmonies wash over us like gentle lapping waves at a beach, while we catch up with what's been happening in our lives.

Once upon a time, Nancy and I would have talked about our weight gains or losses, our unacceptably "fat" thighs or stomachs, or the latest miracle diet plan. But we no longer spend our days preoccupied by dieting, because we know how to keep excess pounds off without struggle and sacrifice.

Now, instead, I talk with Nancy about my challenging and fascinating job and about the everyday joys and trials of family life. Nancy lives in New York and is a successful magazine executive, and like me, she has more important things in her life than food and body preoccupation: her study of language, her friends, her children.

We listen to the music and talk about the fellow travelers we've met or read about on our journey. Some of us are healthy and can laugh at our memories of dieting, even though the pain will never be forgotten. Others still struggle, caught up in a battle with their bodies, continuing to believe that dieting is the key to thinness, acceptance, love, and success. Trapped in the cultural myth that starvation will set them free, these "normal" dieters suffer the unending misery of food restriction and body dissatisfaction. But they are more fortunate than others who died for the cause of thinness, victims of eating disorders that stole their spirits and then their lives.

As we talk, we realize how lucky we are to be survivors of this war on our bodies—because it is nothing less than a war and one that continues, year after year, to claim millions of victims.

The steps to my healing were long and hard, in part because few professionals were available to help me. Most doctors have little understanding of why women (and many men) try diet after diet, why dieting doesn't work, or how to help a person caught in the grip of repetitive dieting or overeating and longing to escape.

Moreover, few professionals know that *overweight people can lose weight— and they can lose it without dieting.* As you know if you've made the rounds of doctors, many believe (a) that weight loss is simply a matter of dieting and (b) that overweight people simply don't try hard enough to lose weight. They don't understand the counterproductive effects of dieting, the physical and emotional toll that dieting takes, or the state-of-the-art medical literature showing that permanent weight loss is possible—but *only* through nondieting techniques.

For these reasons I've spent much of my professional career studying food preoccupations and designing a program to help men and women free themselves from their crippling effects and lose weight safely and permanently. My techniques, based on my own healing and on my successful efforts to help others, are based on an understanding of the complex biological, cultural, and psychological reasons why we become caught in an endless cycle of dieting, too terrified to escape and too tired to continue.

Although I began this book with my own story, it's important to emphasize that the problems that people with "food fear" experience are universal, whether their preoccupation takes the form of eating disorders or compulsive overeating or remains at the "normal" level of yo-yo dieting. In conducting classes and workshops for psychiatrists, medical students, and other health professionals, I'm consistently struck by how many fail to appreciate the devastating effects of *any* level of "food fear." But food is so central to our lives that those of us caught in the web of chronic dieting can identify with others, whether their food preoccupations are milder or more severe.

The four-times-a-year dieter who hates her own body, the overweight woman who hides cookies in the clothes hamper and eats them in secret, the anorexic who puts her life at risk, and the bulimic who binges and purges all suffer from the consequence of debilitating food and body preoccupations. The forty-five-year-old woman who dreads her son's wedding because she "looks fat" in her dress, the twenty-year-old gay man who fears losing his partner if he gains ten pounds, and the teenager who gives up dinner because her boyfriend says she's "getting hippy" all will recognize themselves in this book.

The victims of food and body preoccupation come in all sizes and shapes. Some of us maintain a healthy weight, but we struggle constantly, and our issues with food cause incredible tension in our lives. Many of us are overweight, because the very act of dieting forces our bodies to gain, not lose, weight. Some of us are dangerously gaunt, because we've bought into the myth that there is no such thing as "too thin." And some of us are very large in spite of constant yo-yo dieting, because society's scorn drives us to food—seemingly both our best friend and our worst foe—for comfort.

We are all sisters and brothers, struggling, suffering, and missing out on the joys of life, and there are more of us than you can imagine—all deluded by the myth that dieting will make us thin and set us free. But, as I'll explain in the next chapter, nothing could be farther from the truth. You *can* have the sexy, beautiful body you deserve—but you won't get it by dieting.

Diets Cause Weight Loss: Reality or Myth?

"[T]he diet messiahs have one overriding similarity. They are united in their failure to arrest the spread of fat. Quite simply, if any of their prescriptions fulfilled their promises, we would all be saved. But they don't, and we aren't."

Dale M. Atrens, Ph.D.[1]

YOU *CAN* LOSE your excess pounds. You *can* look great in your clothes, feel sexy and fit, and keep unwanted pounds off forever. But there's a powerful enemy standing in the way of your success, and you need to conquer that enemy before you can lose weight for real and for good.

That enemy—the one you've always been told is your best friend—is dieting. You're told that dieting is the only path to weight loss, that it's safe, and that it's a scientifically proven way to conquer your weight problem. But these "facts" are untrue.

Dieting Causes Weight Loss? A False Belief

As I write this, eighty million Americas are counting carbohydrates, cutting calories, avoiding sugar, eating Jenny Craig meals, or living on cabbage soup or canned weight-loss shakes. Glossy women's magazines, TV fitness gurus, weight-loss centers, and diet book authors tell us that all of this self-denial and sacrifice is worthwhile—that diets work and that if we only spend a little more money, invest a little more time, exhibit a little more willpower, the perfect body is within our reach.

Their message is clear: if you're not a size 6, it's your fault. You're weak. You didn't try hard enough. You're a quitter.

It's in the diet industry's best interest, of course, to tell you this. Promoters of diet products earn millions of dollars each year, simply by preying on desperate dieters who believe their lives will change forever if they can lose weight. But as a medical doctor who has studied dieting extensively (and, perhaps more significantly, experienced dieting firsthand), I know that the saddest thing about all of our starvation and self-deprivation is this:

It's all for nothing.

In fact, for most people dieting is worse than useless. Somewhere between 95 and 98 percent of dieters fail to keep any weight off permanently, but sadder still, many wind up *gaining* weight with each diet. (Perhaps that's why major diet programs aren't interested in having their results analyzed scientifically.[2]) We spend $30 billion a year on diet products, programs, pills, and foods, and almost none of us loses weight permanently as a result.

Of course, that's not what the people who run the diet programs and write the diet books will tell you. Laura Fraser, author of *Losing It: False Hopes and Fat Profits in the Diet Industry*, says, "The diet industry is a sort of perfect business because it is the only business in the world where it fails 95 percent of the time and blames the consumer. I mean, if you bought lightbulbs and they went out 95 percent of the time, they wouldn't say, 'Well, you are not screwing your lightbulbs in right.' "[3]

I'm reminded of the word *delusion*, which in psychiatry is defined as "a fixed false belief." I see a nation of people running themselves ragged, spending more money on weight-loss products than some countries spend on their national budgets, because of our delusion that dieting is the key to weight loss—if only we can stop failing at it.

But in reality we haven't failed at dieting—*dieting has failed us*. That's why almost every miraculous success story you read in ads for Jenny Craig or Nutri/System says, in fine print at the bottom, "results not typical." (A more honest disclaimer for those I-lost-eighty-pounds-in-six-months stories would be "results almost unheard of.") A tiny number of lucky people, of course, do succeed in losing weight on a diet and keeping it off—but for every one of them there are fifty people who try every bit as hard, with no success. Saying that dieting is a successful technique is much like saying that surgery for pancreatic cancer is a rousing success because it cures two or three of every hundred patients—or like saying that playing the lottery is a wise financial strategy because two or three of every hundred people actually win more money than they lose.

With millions of people suffering from the effects of failed diets, we should find strength in our numbers—the strength to say that our lives are too valuable to waste in an endless, unsuccessful battle with food. Unfortunately, the diet industry, abetted by a culture that teaches us to value dangerously distorted body images (see Chapter 3), has succeeded beyond its wildest dreams in convincing us that we are failures if we look, feel, or eat like normal people. We are brainwashed to believe that a woman with a slightly rounded belly is grotesque, that a man without washboard abs is "soft" and weak, that a teenage girl in size-10 jeans is fat. And we are brainwashed to believe that there is only one path to personal fulfillment and an ideal body: constant dieting, constant sacrifice, constant denial. It's a lie—one that causes us enormous suffering, guilt, and shame and offers us no reward and no escape.

If you are still playing the diet game, the most important step you must take to achieve lasting weight loss is to stop believing this lie. *You can't win at dieting, no matter how hard you try.*

Before I explain why, it's important to understand just what a diet is. By dieting, I mean any eating pattern that entails replacing internally driven, hunger-driven eating with externally controlled eating. Obviously, if you're counting calories or drinking Slim-Fast every day instead of eating lunch, that's a diet. But it's also a diet if you tell yourself you can't eat a dessert or snack when you're hungry—or if you restrict yourself to artificial sweeteners, forbid yourself to put your favorite dressing on your salad, or deny yourself certain foods because they're "bad." And it's a diet if a doctor says "Eat whatever you want, but just eat half as much as usual" or "Eat whatever you want, as long as it's healthy food." In short, if you're not eating what you like, when you're hungry for it, you're dieting.

Why does virtually every diet fail? Three reasons. One is that when you diet, your body outsmarts you. The second is that when you diet, you cause a disconnection between your sense of hunger and eating, and that guarantees that you will fail at dieting—unless you diet to the point of risking your life. And the third is that while almost everyone can have an attractive, healthy body, most bodies simply can't be reshaped to look like Brad Pitt's or Cindy Crawford's.

Your Body Is Smarter Than Your Diet

"I just don't have enough willpower." "I'm weak." "I just can't control myself." We find plenty of reasons to blame ourselves, even to hate ourselves, each time we fail at a diet. But the first and most important thing you need to know if you've failed at dieting is that *it's not your fault*. It's not because you're weak or out of control or lack willpower. In reality diets don't work because your body is designed to survive—and survival, for most of the thousands of years we've been evolving, has meant not starving.

Your body expects you to eat enough food each day to keep it healthy, and when you cut down, it hits the panic button. First it starts burning muscle to create more energy. It also turns down your metabolism, the rate at which its internal "factories" burn calories to create energy. To make matters even worse, your body reacts to a diet by increasing the release of enzymes that enable it to store more fat as protection against starvation. In short, the less you eat, the more fat your body attempts to pile on.

Unfortunately, your body is very efficient at playing this game. In a study that won't surprise most dieters, Rudolph Leibel and colleagues gave volunteers (some overweight and others not) calorie-controlled liquid meals for three months and then either upped their calorie intake or decreased it.[4] When the subjects ate fewer calories and began losing weight (whether they initially were overweight or not), the researchers say, "It seemed to set off a bunch of metabolic alarms." The result: the bodies of the people who were losing weight on the lower-calorie diet started burning calories *15 percent more slowly* than before. (Interestingly, the converse was true as well: people who gained weight quickly had trouble keeping it on.)

The researchers concluded that when people gain or lose a great deal of weight quickly, the body compensates by changing energy use—and these changes "oppose the maintenance of a body weight that is different from the usual weight." That means, simply, that if you drastically cut your calories, your body will respond drastically in turn. You'll burn fewer calories, have less energy, feel worse, and, in the long run, fail to lose weight.

Even so, you may succeed temporarily when you diet. Perhaps you'll lose ten or even twenty pounds, mostly water weight or muscle. But your body will keep sending out urgent signals—"Starving! Eat! Now!"—and eventually you'll either binge or give up the diet and go back to your normal eating patterns. In fact you'll probably have even more cravings for fattening foods when you go off a diet, because that's another trick your body pulls: when you starve, it increases your desire for high-calorie foods that put on pounds.

(Again, this makes sense from an evolutionary standpoint. A starving man or woman may die, and a starving woman can't bear healthy children. So our bodies, and particularly women's, are designed to fight starvation in every possible way, from hoarding fat to making us crave cheese pizza and butter pecan ice cream when we're dieting.)

The leader of your body's battle against dieting is your hypothalamus, a small area of your brain that helps regulate everything from sex drive to stress reactions. Among its many jobs, the hypothalamus appears to act a little like a fat thermostat, regulating your biochemistry to maintain your weight at what it believes to be the right level.

The hypothalamus appears to determine your set point—that is, the weight at which it wants you to stay—and then fights tooth and nail to keep you at that weight. (Another current theory is that you have a "settling point," determined by a combination of your genes and your environment. The end result, unfortunately, appears to be the same: by the time you're an adult, your body has decided what weight is right for you and will go to great lengths to maintain that weight.) This is why low-carb or starvation diets that take off the first twenty or thirty pounds with such spectacular success almost always fail, just as spectacularly, a few weeks or months later.

This is depressing enough—but if you're a woman, there's even more bad news about dieting. One important change that occurs when you diet, if you're female (but possibly not if you're male) is that your levels of tryptophan drop.[5] That's bad, because tryptophan, an amino acid, is the building block of a brain chemical called *serotonin*. You've probably heard of serotonin: it's the brain chemical that Prozac and some other antidepressants affect and a chemical that's often altered in people who are depressed. (This suggests one reason why dieting can make you depressed, a topic I'll discuss later.) High serotonin levels help your brain decide that you're satiated—that is, full and contented—after you eat enough carbohydrates. If your serotonin levels plummet as a result of a drop in your tryptophan levels, then you're likely to crave cake, mashed potatoes, and other high-carbohydrate foods.

In short, your body does everything it can to sabotage a diet, and it's almost always successful. Moreover, once you go off a diet, you'll almost always gain back all the weight you've lost, and sometimes you'll gain back more. Why? Because dieting lowered your metabolism, and your body learned to survive on fewer calories. When you start eating again, even if you stick to a regular calorie intake, your body will initially store up pounds—not the pounds of muscle you lost but *fat* pounds. Chronic dieting, in addition to reducing the muscle you need, can actually increase your body fat from 25 percent to 35 to 40 percent over time. The end result of all your dieting efforts: more fat, not less.

Some diets promise that if you eat certain foods or food combinations, you'll somehow keep your metabolism high and lose weight permanently. However, as a physician, I can tell you that in my opinion, these claims are untrue. While almost any diet will help you take off a few pounds fast, no highly restrictive, unnatural diet will keep them off permanently for the overwhelming majority of people.

Ignoring Your Body's Messages Won't Work

Diets don't work for another reason: it's dangerous to stop listening to your body. Yet that's exactly what you do every time you starve yourself.

Imagine what would happen if you ignored your body when it told you, "I need to go to the bathroom" or "I need to sleep" or "I'm dehydrated—I need water" or "I'm very cold—I need warm clothes" or "Ouch! Move your hand—that stove is hot!"

Obviously, you don't do any of these things—at least not on a regular basis. More important, you don't feel guilty about listening to your body when it sends you these messages. You don't feel guilty if you move your hand away from a hot stove. You don't agonize morally over whether or not you should go to the bathroom. You don't worry about whether it's a sign of weakness to stop at a drinking fountain. You don't try to go for weeks without sleeping and tell yourself if you fail, "I'm just so weak." And if you're too cold, you dress appropriately. You don't say to yourself, "You're such a failure—why can't you handle a little frostbite?"

Yet when it comes to food, you ignore your body's warnings all the time. When you're dieting, and your body says, "I'm starving—feed me," you don't heed that message. Instead you say, "I can't eat now." You label your appetite as bad or weak, and you pretend that you can make it go away.

An odd (and very destructive) thing happens when your eating is no longer hunger driven, but instead becomes diet driven. When you're forced to follow an artificial eating schedule, you decouple your appetite from your eating. That means that you don't eat when you're hungry, but *it also means that you binge or graze when you are not hungry.*

"Chronic dieters do not compensate [for eating high-calorie foods] by minimizing further eating, as non-dieters do after eating a large amount," researchers Janet Polivy and C. Peter Herman say. "Instead, dieters appear to become disinhibited; after being preloaded with fattening food, they eat more than similarly treated non-dieters or than dieters who have not [broken] their diets."

As I explained earlier, this is partly a biological response, because your body wants you to eat high-fat foods when it's starving. However, it's also a psychological response. As Polivy and Herman note, dieters who think they've eaten "bad" high-calorie foods will continue to binge on other "bad" foods at hand—even if the food that began the binge was really low in calories. Why? Because dieting makes forbidden foods seem compelling and simultaneously trains you to believe that you have no willpower in the absence of external controls. The result: when you finally rebel against these external controls, and give in to the urge to eat "bad" foods, you eat until you literally are sickened, both physically and emotionally, by your bingeing.

Dieters are also more likely than nondieters to binge or graze when they're upset, when they're drinking, or when they're sick. Bingeing and grazing temporarily soothe both physical and emotional starvation, but at a high price: each binge or grazing episode makes the dieter feel more and more helpless and out of control, leading to a vicious circle of intensified dieting and increased bingeing. It's a perfect recipe for weight gain and self-hatred.

Do You Suffer from Binge-Eating Disorder?

Even many people who don't diet feel out of control in their relationship with food. Surveys indicate that at any given time up to 5 percent of Americans binge frequently and severely enough to receive a
diagnosis of mental disorder. Among the symptoms of severe binge-
eating disorder:

- You experience recurrent episodes of "binge" eating—that is,
  eating a very large amount of food and feeling as though you're
  out of control and can't stop eating.
- Your binge-eating episodes are associated with at least three of
  the following: eating more rapidly than normal; eating until you
  feel physically uncomfortable; eating large amounts of food
  when you are not physically hungry; eating alone because you
  are embarrassed by the amount of food you're eating; or feeling
  disgusted, depressed, or guilty after a binge.
- You feel very distressed, after and between binges, about your
  binge eating.

Binge eating and bulimia (which I'll discuss shortly) are close
cousins. The main difference is that binge eaters don't vomit, use laxatives, or engage in other inappropriate compensatory behaviors such
as fasting or excessive exercise to compensate for their eating, so they
often gain a great deal of weight.

Of course, a handful of people—that supposedly lucky 5 percent—do
succeed at overriding their body's needs and maintaining the weight they've
reached on a diet. But most do so only by sacrificing, forever, a relaxed and
normal relationship with food. Every food-related family tradition becomes
an inner conflict ("How do I tell my mother I can't eat her hamantaschen?"),
and every special occasion becomes a crisis ("Can I sit through the whole
wedding dinner without eating 'bad' food?"). Even a simple restaurant meal

or a box of Valentine's Day candy is transformed into a danger to be avoided, a temptation to be resisted. We never realize how large a role food plays in our heritage, our family life, our holidays, and our celebrations, until we attempt to reduce eating to a mechanical, calories-in, calories-out process.

You're Stuck with Your Genes

We diet in a desperate search for the Holy Grail: the one perfect body we believe is inside us, masked by unsightly and repulsive fat and just waiting to be freed. But eventually we learn that no matter how much we diet, we'll never, ever look like Kate Moss or Pierce Brosnan.

Why? Because very slender people generally come from very slender families, and most of the rest of us don't. We can't starve away our bones (and yes, most of us *are* big-boned compared to Kate Moss). We can't alter the fact that our bodies tend to deposit fat in the same spots as our mothers' or fathers' bodies. And, just as we can't make our boobs magically grow into watermelons, we can't make our thighs shrink to pencils if our genes say "no way."

That *doesn't* mean, however, that you're doomed to be overweight. In fact very few people are genetically hardwired to be obese (although a handful are, just as a few people are very tall). It does mean, however, that you probably can't reach Ally McBeal–like gauntness by any means short of divine intervention. What you can do, as I'll explain in this book, is attain the right weight and figure for *you*. Odds are you won't look like a *Vogue* model, but you'll have a beautiful, healthy, sexy body.

Dieting, however, isn't the way to reach that goal. As I've explained, each time you diet, you lose muscle and gain back fat. Thus each diet you go on will actually leave you another step farther away from looking as good as you can.

A Dangerous Obsession

If dieting just wasted your time, it would be bad enough. But dieting is also very dangerous—not just for anorexics and bulimics but also for average, everyday dieters. Typical yo-yo dieting (what medical professionals call *weight cycling*) doesn't just damage your self-esteem; it can damage your body as well. That's why, unlike most doctors who call dieting a healthy activity, I call it what it really is: *a disease*.

How does dieting jeopardize your health? Here's a short list.

• **Dieting hurts your heart and cardiovascular system.** Studies of large groups of people show that yo-yo dieting can increase your risk of death from cardiovascular disease.[6] Why? One recent study found that yo-yo dieting significantly lowers levels of the "good" cholesterol HDL-C in women,[7] and another study of rats showed that weight cycling disrupts levels of serum cholesterol, triglycerides, glucose, and insulin in ways that could increase heart disease risk.[8] Yo-yo dieting is dangerous for men's hearts as well as women's: one study found that men who experience at least one cycle of major weight loss and regain are at increased risk of death from cardiovascular disease compared to men who steadily gain weight or those whose weight remains stable.[9]

• **Dieting can break your bones.** Yo-yo dieting reduces your bone mass and increases your risk of hip fractures.[10] Because we stockpile bone mass during childhood and early adulthood, it's particularly dangerous for pre-teens, teens, and young adults to diet.

• **Dieting can increase your risk of gallstones.** Middle-aged women are especially prone to this painful and sometimes dangerous medical problem, which often requires major surgery called a *cholecystectomy*. According to a recent study, "the risk for cholecystectomy associated with weight cycling [is] substantial, independent of attained relative body weight."[11] For years, doctors told patients that the highest-risk group for gallstones is "fat, female, and forty," but we're learning that being overweight may be less risky than weight cycling.

• **Dieting can affect your immune system.** When you reduce your calorie consumption drastically, you also dramatically reduce the numbers of disease-fighting cells in your body,[12] putting you at increased risk for infections and possibly even cancer.

• **Dieting causes changes in the breast.** Two recent studies link weight cycling to DNA damage or abnormal cell changes in breast tissue, meaning that yo-yo dieting may increase a woman's risk of breast cancer.[13]

• **Dieting may increase a woman's risk of having a hysterectomy.** It sounds strange, but research indicates that yo-yo dieting is strongly linked to menstrual problems serious enough to require removal of the uterus.[14]

• **Dieting can ruin your teeth.** Extreme dieting can deprive you of the calcium you need to have strong, healthy teeth. If you purge after bingeing, the stomach acids you bring up can cause the enamel on your teeth to erode. Chronic purging can lead to cavities, tooth staining, and even the necessity for tooth removal.

• **Dieting makes you physically weak.** Study after study reports that physical fatigue is one of the primary side effects of dieting.

• **Dieting is bad for your mental health.** I'll talk later about how dieting can make you feel bad about yourself. But it can also make your *brain* feel bad. As I mentioned, women who diet have reduced levels of tryptophan, the building block of the brain chemical serotonin—and low serotonin levels are linked to depression, hostility, impulsive behavior, obsessive-compulsive behavior, and even an increased risk of suicide.

In addition, dieting appears to make you less smart—no kidding. A recent study found that women had slower reaction times, exhibited poorer immediate recall of words, and were less vigilant on cognitive tests when they were dieting than when they weren't.[15]

• **Dieting can put you at risk for alcohol abuse.** Canadian researchers evaluated the dieting behaviors and alcohol use of nearly two hundred female university students. They report that levels of food restraint correlated strongly with how much the women drank and how often they engaged in "binge drinking." "Chronic dieting," the researchers say, "appears to be related to a relatively heavy drinking pattern that can be characterized as potentially risky."[16]

That's a frightening list, and it doesn't even include the dangers posed by weight-loss drugs. We all remember fen-phen, the diet pill that was the craze of the late 1990s before we learned that it could irreversibly damage heart valves. Ephedra, an herbal supplement touted as a weight-loss drug, also led to the deaths of several dieters. New evidence links excessive laxative use, common in bulimics, anorexics, and even "normal" dieters, to long-term pancreatic damage.[17] And millions of people who worry about their weight continue to take over-the-counter diet drugs containing artificial stimulants that can cause sleeplessness, anxiety, and heart irregularities.

Of course being overweight is also a serious health issue. Unlike some other experts, I'm not going to try to convince you that it's OK, medically speaking, to weigh three or four hundred pounds. It's not, because being very overweight increases your chances of suffering from diabetes, sleep apnea, heart disease, and even some forms of cancer. It seems unfair, I know: you're at risk if you're carrying around extra pounds, but you're at risk if you try to lose them by dieting.

In reality, however, there *is* a solution. Fortunately, as I'll explain later, you can reach your ideal weight *without dieting* and without potentially dangerous drugs. You *can* have the best of both worlds: a healthy, attractive body and eating habits that allow you to be both healthy and comfortable with food. My goal, in talking about the dangers of dieting, is not to frighten you, but to encourage you to seek a better way to improve your health—an approach that will keep you looking and feeling great for the rest of your life.

When Dieting Takes a Deadly Turn

Clearly, even typical dieting is hazardous to your health. For millions of people, however, dieting is also the first step in a tragic spiral into dangerous or even deadly eating disorders. It sounds obvious to say that dieting leads to eating disorders; after all, it's almost impossible to become anorexic if you never start on a diet. But there's more to it than that: as I'll explain, chronic dieting actually *changes you biologically and psychologically* in ways that make you a target for eating disorders.

These disorders are an epidemic in Western societies, with at least five of every hundred young women suffering from anorexia or bulimia. Thousands of teens and young women die of anorexia each decade, and millions of other anorexics and bulimics require medical treatment for premature osteoporosis, heart disease, and other crippling medical disorders.

These victims, however, are just the tip of a huge iceberg. In reality, the number of individuals with eating disorders is tremendously underreported, because of the secrecy and shame associated with anorexia and bulimia. In addition, the majority of eating disorders that are reported are those classifiable according to the *Diagnostic and Statistical Manual of Mental Disorders (DSM-IV)*, the official manual of mental health disorders. But the *DSM* definitions of eating disorders exclude huge numbers of women and growing numbers of men who—while they may not look like the starving children in Oxfam posters or bear scars on their hands from vomited stomach acids—

still suffer terribly because their preoccupation with thinness restricts their lives and cripples them emotionally.

If the definition of eating disorders is extended to include these subclinical sufferers, millions of additional women, and thousands of men, qualify as eating disordered. These silent victims, as Carol Bloom and Laura Kogel note, "are not totally 'taken over' by their symptoms and obsessions, yet they are involved with a riveting preoccupation, an encapsulated piece of 'madness' that moves from background to foreground, depending on triggers in their inner and/or outer life."[18] Whether we label this level of preoccupation as an "eating disorder not otherwise specified" (see *DSM* definitions of eating disorders in the sidebar[19]) or simply as extreme dieting, the consequences to its sufferers are devastating.

Do You Have an Eating Disorder?

The following are textbook symptoms of eating disorders. However, it's important to realize that *even if you suffer from only a few of these symptoms, you may suffer from subclinical eating disorder that is severely endangering your mental along with your physical health.*

The Anorexic Individual

- fails to maintain a minimum body weight (for example, 85 percent of expected weight for height and age)
- has an intense fear of becoming fat, despite being underweight
- has a distorted body image and believes that he or she is overweight
- bases his or her self-esteem on weight or shape
- denies the seriousness of being underweight
- if female, has missed at least three consecutive periods (or has periods only when taking hormones)

(continued)

There are two primary types of anorexia:

Binge-Eating/Purging Type. Involves purging (vomiting or use of laxatives or diuretics) and/or binge eating.

Restricting Type. Involves severe restriction of food intake but does not involve bingeing or purging during an anorectic episode.

The Bulimic Individual

- repeatedly eats in binges; during these episodes, the bulimic consumes much more food than is normal and feels that his or her eating is out of control
- repeatedly uses fasting, self-induced vomiting, excessive exercise, or abuse of laxatives, diuretics, or other drugs in order to lose weight
- experiences binge eating and purging at least twice a week
- bases his or her self-esteem primarily on weight and body shape
- is not anorexic. Most bulimics are of average weight.

There are two primary types of bulimia:

Purging Type: Involves frequent vomiting or use of diuretics or laxatives. This is the more well-known type.

Nonpurging Type: Involves excessive fasting or exercise, but does not generally involve vomiting or use of diuretics or laxatives.

Eating Disorder Not Otherwise Specified

Psychiatrists use this definition to describe people who do not meet the full criteria for an eating disorder but who exhibit food and weight preoccupations serious enough to interfere with their daily lives and mental health. These are men and women who might "pass for normal" but in fact spend much of their lives in a state of intense anxiety about their weight and eating—an anxiety that prevents them from enjoying life and relationships. Many of the people I counsel fall into this category.

Reprinted with permission from the *Diagnostic and Statistical Manual of Mental Disorders, Fourth Edition, Text Revision.* Copyright 2000 American Psychiatric Association.

It's true that some people are more vulnerable to eating disorders than others, but if you believe you're not at risk, think again. Millions of women in America are bulimic or anorexic, and these disorders strike all categories of women: athletes, intellectuals, married women, single women, girls entering puberty, and even women entering menopause. While genes, personality, and personal experiences can affect the risk of developing an eating disorder, it's clear that few women can honestly say, "It can't happen to me." Males, too, particularly athletes and gay men, are increasingly falling prey to both anorexia and bulimia.

Moreover, almost all anorexics and bulimics begin as typical dieters, and many of the distorted beliefs associated with anorexia and bulimia are common among dieters in general. The messages of our fat-phobic society translate, all too easily, into compulsive dieting—and, frequently, from dieting into life-threatening eating disorders.

But if dieting makes us psychologically vulnerable to eating disorders, it also makes us biologically vulnerable. Remember what I said about dieting throwing your brain chemistry off? There's strong evidence that this dysregulation of brain chemicals, particularly serotonin, can set a dieter on the road to eating disorders.

As I've mentioned, if you're a woman, dieting reduces your plasma levels of tryptophan, the building block of the brain chemical serotonin. Recently a group of researchers studied the effects of tryptophan depletion on two groups of women: recovering bulimics and women with no history of eating disorders. The researchers asked the women to drink either a balanced amino acid mixture or a mixture lacking tryptophan. (None of the women knew which type of mixture they were drinking or the purpose of the study.)

The results: when women with a history of bulimia drank the tryptophan-depleted drink, they experienced "significant lowering of mood, increases in ratings of body image concern, and subjective loss of control of eating." The researchers conclude that chronic depletion of tryptophan "may be one of the mechanisms whereby persistent dieting can lead to the development of eating disorders in vulnerable individuals."[20]

The more we learn, the clearer it becomes that dieting is often the first step, both mentally and physically, on the road to eating disorders. Are you vulnerable? Very possibly, if you're a frequent or compulsive dieter. There's no such thing as being "too smart" to develop an eating disorder, as proven by the fact that anorexia and bulimia are rampant on college campuses. And there's no such thing as being "too successful" to develop an eating disorder—just ask the dozens of famous skaters, gymnasts, and dancers who spend their days garnering applause and endorsements and their nights hunched over toilets vomiting.

The only effective means of protecting yourself from developing an eating disorder is to avoid diets that push you, both psychologically and biologically, toward a destructive new level of food restriction and weight preoccupation. That's yet another reason to say "no" to diets and say "yes" to healthy, diet-free weight loss. But even if you're not worried about eating disorders, you need to recognize that diets are both counterproductive and dangerous.

The Bottom Line: Diets Are Self-Defeating

Clearly the weight-loss gurus who crank out new miracle diets every other day aren't telling you about the medical literature on dieting. They aren't telling you that diets almost always fail. They aren't telling you that diets replace muscle with fat and often make you *gain* weight. They aren't showing you the evidence that dieting is bad for your body, putting you at risk for heart disease, depression, and osteoporosis. And they aren't telling you that for many people, dieting is the first step toward dangerous or even fatal eating disorders.

The diet pushers don't have to tell you these facts because it's not their goal to make you attractive, healthy, or happy. It's their goal to get rich.

Unfortunately, they succeed all too well at this goal. Even when diets fail us time after time after time, we continue to try every new weight-loss plan, desperately believing, "This is the one." Our endless search for the Holy Grail of a weight-loss miracle keeps us trapped, unaware that the only true way to lose weight—and keep it off, without deprivation and sacrifice—is to *stop dieting and start working with, not against, our bodies.*

Jean-Paul Deslypere, University of Ghent professor of human nutrition, says, "Dieting may be the major cause of obesity." The path to freedom from being overweight, conversely, begins with two words: I quit. The day you quit dieting is the first day that you take a positive step toward a beautiful, sexy, healthy body and freedom—forever—from "food fear."

To take that step, however, you need to face one more enemy. That enemy, the one that drove you to endless dieting in the first place, is a culture that tells you, every hour of every day, that you'll never be happy, successful, or loved unless you're impossibly and even dangerously thin.

America's Culture of Food Fear

Why Do We Diet When Dieting Doesn't Work?

"Virtually all [fashion] magazines send one clear message: Your body is a mess."

Barbara Dafoe Whitehead[1]

THE STEPS IN this book will teach you how to lose your excess pounds and enable you to become fit, sexy, and happy in your body. But if you're looking for a fitness plan to turn you into a Calvin Klein model, you're reading the wrong book. That's because my goal is to make you attractive and healthy—not to make you sick and sad.

To obtain the perfect body for you, you must first realize that there is no single standard of perfection—just as there is no single "correct" color for a flower or "correct" design for a snowflake. However, this can be a difficult concept to grasp fully in a culture that considers anyone larger than a size 8 to be "too big" and that values unnatural bodies over healthy ones.

In the fall of 1987, I stood on a New York sidewalk watching the West Indian Day Parade on Eastern Parkway.

Sensual music pulsed as dozens and dozens of women swirled down the street in colorful, vibrant, wild attire—feathers, beaded loincloths, sequins, huge headdresses, scarlet and emerald bandana tops baring their cleavage and their navels. They danced the length of the parkway, reveling in the movement, the beat of the music, and their bodies.

They had wide hips, swinging breasts, rounded bellies, and most weighed more than 140 pounds. They were beautiful and sexy, and they knew it.

These women loved their bodies and rejoiced in their femininity, because their culture admired the curve of their breasts and the swell of their rounded thighs and buttocks. My world, conversely, told me to look like a starving waif. It told me that at 5'8" and 145 pounds I was too big to be proud of my body, much less flaunt it openly on a New York street. It told me to hide my rounded breasts and hips under baggy sweats and to feel shame if I allowed myself to gain a pound.

Maybe, I realized, as the dancers passed by proudly, my world was wrong.

If dieting doesn't work, why do you do it—and why do you *keep* doing it, in spite of failure after failure?

One answer is that if you're an American, your culture tells you, in every way it can, to hate your body. It also tells you that your body is, as psychology professor Ruth Striegel-Moore says, "infinitely malleable" and that with enough willpower and money you can remold it into any shape you desire. Moreover, it creates standards of beauty that are unnatural, dangerous, and, for most of us, completely unattainable.

Don't get me wrong: you *can* lose weight, if you're overweight, and attain a slimmer, healthier body. But if you believe that happiness and beauty are only for size-2 women or men in size-32 jeans, then you will be doomed to unhappiness by the cultural myths you've bought into. Before you can gain the courage to stop your endless cycle of dieting, and be happy in the healthy body that's perfect for *you*, you need to understand just how powerful and destructive these cultural influences are and why, as a man or woman in modern-day America, you're uniquely vulnerable to them.

What's Your "Ideal" Body?

As a first step toward this understanding, do this simple exercise. Close your eyes for a moment and visualize your ideal body. Picture exactly how you should look: how large your breasts (or your chest, if you're a man) should be, what size and shape your hips and buns should be, how much you should weigh.

If you're a woman, the body you've pictured is probably a size 6, weighs around 110 pounds, and has C-cup breasts, a flat stomach, a tiny round bottom, and boyish thighs. If you're a man, your ideal body most likely has a V-shaped torso, weighs about 175 pounds, and has washboard abs, a thirty-one-inch waist, a rock-hard little butt, and a muscular chest and thighs.

Now, ask yourself a simple question:

Who told you that's the perfect body?

If your response is "my mother" or "my girlfriend" or "my husband," then let's revise the question a little:

Who told *them* that's the perfect body?

These may seem like strange questions. After all, you just "know" that you're too fat, too "jiggly," too bottom-heavy, or too wide in the waist. And you just "know" that the models on the covers of the magazines in the grocery line are perfect.

But *how* do you know?

The answer, in large part, is that your culture tells you so. Your culture tells you how you to dress and behave, what color to paint your fingernails, how wide your power ties should be, even what's moral and immoral. And when it comes to bodies, your culture tells you who is beautiful and who isn't.

Many of your ideas about beauty come from your parents, friends, neighbors, teachers, co-workers, and people you date or marry. Still others come from pictures you see in museums, conversations you hear at the mall, and books. But in today's society we've granted one particular group of people the ultimate authority to dictate our ideals of beauty. These people, more than any others, define the perfection you struggle every day to achieve. They tell you how long your hair should be, how big your breasts should be, how small your nose must be, even how "ethnic" you're allowed to look. And they bombard you with constant messages, every hour of every day, telling you just how far you are from attaining the standards they've set.

I'm talking, of course, about the media and Madison Avenue. Over the course of your life, you'll probably spend more than seven years' worth of time watching TV and see nearly two million TV commercials. In addition, you'll see thousands of movies and read nearly twenty thousand magazines containing more than a million ads. And almost every show you watch, every movie you view, and every ad you read will transmit powerful messages about weight or beauty.

To an astonishing extent, Americans swim in a sea of cultural images about beauty, virtually all of which make us feel insecure or ugly if we aren't small-waisted, flat-hipped, tight-bunned, big-haired, and big-chested (but not *too* big-chested). With a few notable exceptions the media present generously endowed people, and particularly women, as the butt of humor, or they refuse to show them at all. One study, for instance, found that 69 percent of female TV characters are thin and only 5 percent are larger than average.[2] Much like African-Americans in the 1950s, who almost never appeared on television except as butlers and maids, the size-12-or-above woman in the twenty-first century is nearly invisible in the world portrayed by TV, movies, magazines, and advertisers.

The media play an increasing role in defining male bodies as well as female bodies, and this new focus on men's appearance is translating into increasing numbers of male dieters and male bulimics and anorexics. Increasingly, men are becoming obsessed with body image, and as many as 10 percent of anorexics are men. Gay men in particular worry about body image, with more than a quarter saying they dislike their bodies, 25 percent reporting that they binge, and more than 10 percent admitting that they vomit to avoid gaining weight.[3]

Straight men, too, are falling under the spell of the "hardbody." A recent issue of *GQ*, for instance, reviewed the top five diet plans and exhorted, "Step away from that cocktail wienie!" One recent body-image study found that 45 percent of men are dissatisfied with their physiques,[4] and plastic surgeon Arnis Freiburg, commenting on the skyrocketing number of men undergoing liposuction—more than 20,000 in 1997, compared to only 6,000 in 1992—says, "The double standard between the sexes is narrowing but may be moving in the wrong direction."[5] (Even ultra-thin Calvin Klein reportedly underwent liposuction in 1996, because he was ashamed of his "love handles."[6]) Another indication of men's growing insecurity: 6 percent of males use dangerous anabolic steroids by the time they're eighteen,[7] and these drugs are used to enhance looks more often than to improve athletic ability.

Men still experience far less "body prejudice" than women, however, because our culture allows them tremendous diversity compared to the unforgiving guidelines for women. (Consider, for instance, the fact that Kelsey Grammer's middle-aged figure drew no comments when he recently became America's highest-paid TV actor—and compare that to the media furor several years ago over the weight of Kirstie Alley, Grammer's former *Cheers* costar and a lovely woman with a typical middle-aged woman's shape, when she landed the starring role in *Veronica's Closet*.) In the film industry, too, men can grow plumper or older and still play leading roles while women can't, a peculiar rule that's led to a slew of movies featuring Sean Connery, Harrison Ford, Jack Nicholson, and other fiftyish or sixtyish actors romancing leading ladies who are barely out of their teens.

In short, this chapter is primarily about women, for the simple reason that it is still women who bear the brunt of the dangerous expectations the media promote about beauty, particularly when it comes to weight. Worse yet, those expectations keep changing—always becoming farther from our grasp. Increasingly, our culture's standards of female beauty, as spelled out by TV, the movies, magazines, and advertisers, are so unrealistic that virtually no normal woman can come close to achieving them.

Thus, unlike most men, women have a tremendous amount of cultural baggage to jettison before they can achieve long-term weight loss. That's because unrealistic expectations push women into unhealthy, counterproductive diets that make them more overweight—not slimmer.

The Ever-Changing "Perfect" Body

If you were a woman living in the 1800s, who would define your standards of beauty? The girl who lived down the street. The town librarian. Your sister-in-law. In short, you'd compare yourself to a handful of neighbors, relatives, and friends, in differing sizes and shapes, none artificially enhanced by silicone or liposuction. These women might strap themselves into tight corsets, pad themselves here and there, and pinch their cheeks to create an artificial glow, but otherwise they'd look like real people.

With the advent of the mass media, however, women now find themselves being compared not just to the girl down the street, but also to the most beautiful (and often surgically enhanced) women in the world. It's no longer good enough to look normal; instead, you need to look like Calista Flockhart or Demi Moore. Moreover, in their eternal striving to be new, radical, and "cutting edge," the media and advertisers keep *changing* our standards of beauty, constantly raising the bar so our goals become ever more unnatural and even bizarre.

Just how arbitrarily do the media and advertisers influence our ideas about beauty—and, in particular, about who's "fat" and who isn't? Only one hundred years ago, America's first lady of the stage, considered to be the greatest beauty of her time, was Lillian Russell, who weighed nearly two hundred pounds. Only fifty years ago, America's sex goddess was Marilyn Monroe, a well-endowed size 12. Yet Russell would be considered obese by today's standards, and philosophy professor Susan Bordo says one of her male students recently commented that Monroe was "a cow." (Moreover, while you can buy copies of Monroe's famous dresses on the Internet today, they're available only in sizes up to 8!)

Similarly, Bordo notes, the bra sizes advertised as "average" in the 1960s are now, only forty years later, advertised as "full-figured" sizes.[8] And driving to work recently, I heard a radio ad encouraging women to audition for modeling jobs. The modeling agency was looking for "plus size" models— which, they explained, meant *size 10* or above.

What happened between now and then? Casting about for new and startling images, advertisers of the 1960s discovered Twiggy—a ninety-pound, 5'8" tall British model—and made her famous. Overnight, a generation of young girls started striving to emulate Twiggy's no-hips, no-boobs, nine-year-old boy look. Twiggy and Jean Shrimpton, another androgynous sixties model, set the stage for four generations of increasingly artificial, unnatural, and unhealthy cultural ideals offered by the media and advertisers.

The skinny trend culminated in the 1990s with "heroin chic," promoted by designer Calvin Klein, in which models looked not only anorexic but actually emaciated and even diseased. Psychologist Liz Dittrich notes that "the average size of idealized woman (as portrayed by models) has become progressively thinner and has stabilized at 13 to 19 percent below physically expected weight."[9] (Some estimates now place the figure at 23 percent.) Today's most popular supermodels include the nearly invisible Trish Goff and Gisele Bundchen, who oddly is billed as heralding a return to the "real woman ideal" although she stands 5'11" and weighs 115 pounds. Television and the movies have followed suit, with the Elizabeth Taylors and Sophia Lorens of the fifties and sixties giving way to the Winona Ryders and Calista Flockharts of the new century. Even children's cartoons have fallen under the spell; as Elizabeth Toledo of the National Organization for Women notes, "Disney's animated female lead characters, such as Pocahontas and the Little Mermaid, are drawn with large breasts, tiny waists, and long slender legs, despite their youthful ages."[10]

In short, America went, in only a hundred years, from idolizing a mature size-18 actress to insisting that its women look like starved child-waifs, only with huge breasts (a look that's been dubbed "boobs on a stick"). Ironically, we've pushed this trend so far, and the ideal body is now so unnatural, that virtually no one—including America's most "perfect" women—can achieve it. As a result, television stars and fashion models, in addition to starving themselves (and often smoking or using prescription or street drugs to keep weight off), undergo painful and demeaning surgeries to increase their chests, suck the fat from their bellies, and sculpt their buttocks.

Thus, the bar is raised even higher for the rest of us: not only must you diet to the point of emaciation, but you must also correct any remaining "problem areas" by going under the knife, filling your chest with balloons, and vacuuming out unwanted pounds.

An Epidemic of Self-Hate

The result of these impossible demands is that by the time we become young adults almost all of us have learned to hate our bodies—because our bodies can't possibly resemble the bodies the media hold up as ideal. While this is true for many men, it's even more true for women. In fact, psychiatrists even have a name for this phenomenon: *normative discontent*. Why "normative"? Because in our society, *it's normal, if you're female, to be unhappy with your body*. Go to a party. What do you hear? Women talking about weight loss, weight gain, past diets, future diets, current diets. Women talking about personal trainers and grueling exercise routines. Women saying, "I'd quit smoking, but I'm afraid of getting fat."

Some women, of course, really are overweight to the point that it endangers their health. What's interesting, however, is that so many women who *aren't* overweight believe that they are. One study by J. Kevin Thompson found that more than 95 percent of women overestimate the size of their bodies, often considerably.[11] Similarly, a survey by *Glamour* magazine found that of the 33,000 women responding, three-quarters considered themselves fat, even though only one-quarter exceeded the weight recommended by experts and 30 percent were *under*weight.[12]

Our phobia of becoming fat—or, more accurately, of being anything other than unnaturally thin—starts earlier and earlier with each passing decade. One survey found that 50 percent of nine-year-old schoolgirls have already been on a diet. The same survey found that 90 percent of seventeen-year-olds were dieting, even though only less than 20 percent of those on a diet were above a healthy weight.[13] And more recently, a study found that five-year-old girls whose weight is above the norm think less of their cognitive abilities and have lower self-esteem than girls of average weight or below. "It was startling," said one of the researchers conducting the study. "If girls are showing these issues at age five, it doesn't look hopeful for what is going to happen to them as teenagers or as young women."[14]

In addition, for the first time in history, the smoking rate of girls now surpasses that of boys,[15] with many of the girls who smoke saying that they took up the habit because they see it as the primary means to lose weight. Harvard researchers say girls are twice as likely to contemplate starting smoking between the ages of nine and fourteen if they are worried about losing weight—meaning that by early puberty our children have learned that it's better to risk death later on than to have normal baby fat right now.[16]

And no wonder! As Michele Humland, a pediatrician who treats eating-disordered adolescents, says, "When kids read the comments about perfectly normal size women like Kate Winslet and Alicia Silverstone being called fat and chubby and being passed over for movie roles, what are they to think? When kids read in *People* magazine that 'plus size' models are 5-foot-8 and 140 pounds—their normal size—what are they to think?"[17]

A few months ago, I watched as a little eight-year-old who'd been swimming in the pool with my daughters weighed herself on the scale at my gym. "I don't want to weigh fifty or a hundred," she said out loud to herself. Studying the reading on the scale anxiously, she sighed and asked me, "What is 50 plus 24?"

I was speechless at first, but then I told her I thought she was a beautiful girl. Watching the desperation and disbelief in her eyes, I saw an eating disorder in the making.

This fear of being "too big" is a terror that most women never lose. As a practicing psychiatrist for more than ten years, I find it striking that in almost every serious psychotherapy I've ever conducted with a woman patient, body shape and food arose as important issues—whether the woman wore a size 20 or a size 2. In fact, as a therapist, I can tell you that it's a myth that extreme thinness brings happiness; instead, it usually brings even greater despair, because maintaining an abnormally thin body is nearly impossible. The closer we get to the elusive goal of model thinness, the harder it gets and the more terrified we become of losing control.

There is no such thing as "thin enough"—no point at which we decide that we're perfect and happy. A case in point: psychotherapists Candace DePuy and Dana Dovitch commented in a recent magazine article, "Did you see the May issue of *Vogue* magazine? Cultural ideal Elizabeth Hurley was on the cover. She is quoted as saying that she is extremely uncomfortable being photographed in a bikini and that she never stands up at a pool! Could there be a more perfect cultural litmus test than this? The woman who walks around in the ideal female body isn't even satisfied herself!"[18] Similarly, 105-pound actress Demi Moore told *Rolling Stone* magazine, "I'm square, I have no waist, and I'm never thin enough, and that's the truth."

There's a scene in the Julia Roberts movie *Notting Hill* in which the characters decide that the one who can tell the saddest story will get the last brownie left over from dessert. Each one tells of a tragedy—unemployment, infertility, the accident that left one paralyzed—but Roberts's character, a famous millionaire actress, comes close to winning the brownie with her sad story: "I've been on a diet every day since I was nineteen, which basically means I've been hungry for a decade." It's a scene that's intended to make the viewer laugh, but most women can identify with it; no matter how successful we are, no matter how beautiful, no matter how rich or lucky, we still feel the deprivation caused by starving ourselves—and we still feel terrified if we *don't* starve ourselves.

Spreading "Food Fear" Around the Globe

Remarkably, the unrealistic images promoted by American television shows are causing body dissatisfaction not just among American men and women but in other societies as well. Harvard researchers studied teenage girls in Nadroga, Fiji, in 1995—when American TV first arrived there—and again in 1998. Initially, only 3 percent of the girls reported vomiting to control their weight. Three years later, 15 percent of them reported this behavior. Girls who watched at least three nights of TV each week were 50 percent more likely to say that they were too fat, and 30 percent more likely to diet, than the girls who didn't watch much TV—even though the TV watchers didn't weigh more than the nonwatchers.

One girl interviewed by the researchers said, "We can see [teenagers] on TV. . . . They are the same ages, but they are working, they are slim and very tall, and they are cute, nice. . . . We want our bodies to become like that. . . . so we try to lose a lot of weight."[19]

Within America, too, cultural groups once nearly immune to food preoccupations and eating disorders (perhaps, in part, because the media refused to depict them at all until the last few decades!) are falling prey to media expectations. *Essence* magazine, a publication aimed primarily at an African-American readership, conducted a large-scale survey on food preoccupation and eating disorders in the 1990s and concluded, "largeness . . . once accepted—even revered—[among Blacks] . . . now carries the same unmistakable stigma as it does among Whites." Similarly, a recent study by Liz Dittrich of more than two hundred junior college women found that 56 percent of African-American women, 58 percent of Latina women, 46 percent of white women, and 43 percent of Asian-American women were trying to lose weight. Dittrich suggests that as women of color become more a part of the cultural mainstream, they increasingly are "pressured to emulate the mainstream image."[20]

To men and women in societies untouched by Western media, in contrast, the "boobs on a stick" image of female perfection seems bizarre. Researchers studying a remote area of Peru, for instance, asked men to pick the ideal female shape from a series of sketches. The men picked a thick-waisted shape, considered overweight by Western standards. Asked to rate a thinner shape, one man declared that it was "pale" and "almost dead." Another called a drawing of a thin, hourglass shape "skinny in the waist" and suggested that its owner "had diarrhea."[21]

The difference between the Peruvian and Western ideals is not which shape each culture prefers, of course—since both ideals overlook the fact that healthy, beautiful women come in all shapes and sizes—but the fact that the Peruvian men at least appreciate a shape that *actually resembles a large percentage of the real women in their culture.* The ideal female body envisioned by the American media, in contrast, cannot be achieved naturally, without starvation or surgery, by more than a tiny percent of women. As an ad by the Body Shop notes, "There are three billion women who don't look like supermodels, and only eight who do."

Why Don't We Just Say "No"?

It's easy (and correct) to criticize American culture, and particularly the media, for perpetrating destructive myths about beauty. But it's important to recognize that while our culture feeds our obsession with thinness, *we've agreed to accept these myths.* After all, cultural stereotypes cannot persist unless we agree to be both victims and accomplices in the starvation and defacement of our bodies. And we do. When our culture says, "You're too fat," even when we're not, we race en masse to diet centers and gyms. When it says, "Your boobs are too small," we spend thousands of dollars packing them with saltwater or silicone. When it says, "Your bodies are ugly," we obediently hide them under baggy sweats. When it says "Starve," we starve and even die.

Why do we allow our culture to define beauty as nothing above a size 6? Largely because women are more vulnerable than men to cultural messages about beauty. Part of the reason is personal: women are more prone to be perfectionists, "pleasers," and harsh self-critics, characteristics that go hand in hand with food preoccupations.

In addition, as Susan Bordo notes, we're trained, early on, to view the male body as functional and active and the female body as aesthetic and decorative. As philosopher John Berger put it, "Men act, and women appear." When counselor Susan Kano asked fifty college students to talk about body satisfaction, she says, the women talked about how they looked while the men talked about their health and their athletic ability. "Women automatically judged their bodies on an ornamental basis," she says, "while men judged their bodies on an instrumental basis."[22] That's why women have put up with corsets, bustles, high heels, and a host of other clothes that made us look beautiful in the eyes of our culture while making it almost impossible for us to function.

We're also trained, as women, to define ourselves by our relationships. If we fail to conform to society's expectations, we may wind up alone—a terrifying idea to women living in a society that denigrates and ridicules "old maids." (I once asked a class of medical students to imagine a forty-five-year-old single male and tell me the words that came to their minds. These second-year medical students replied, "smart," "successful," and "bachelor." I then asked them to picture a forty-five-year-old single woman, and they responded with "spinster" and "ugly.") For centuries women have conformed to painful or even cruel societal rules because they fear risking losing boyfriends or husbands and thus, in their eyes, losing their very identities.

The idea of actually starving ourselves, however, is a new one—and, strangely, one that seems to parallel women's greatest advances as a sex. The first time in American history that thinness became obligatory was during the "flapper" era of the 1920s, when women first shed their constrictive clothes, along with constrictive ideals dictating that women should be modest, quiet, and always subordinate to men. By the 1950s, women were back in their traditional roles as "happy homemakers," and buxom, wide-hipped Marilyn Monroe was our national icon. Then came the revolutionary decade of the sixties, when women achieved sexual freedom and career doors closed for centuries were suddenly flung open. It was a remarkable, empowering time for women—and a time when anorexia and bulimia, once almost unknown, became epidemic. That epidemic continues to grow, seemingly paralleling the gains women are making in the job market, the political arena, and other fields.

It's as if, by declaring ourselves free and capable—able to go to college, become doctors and lawyers, take on roles formerly denied to us—we somehow fear that we are becoming too powerful, even as though we are "taking up too much space." Are we unconsciously reacting by making our bodies frailer, less intimidating, so that we don't threaten men in our new roles? Are we rejecting old cultural roles—our mothers' roles—by looking less maternal, less "housewifely," and more androgynous and muscular? Is being thin a way of sending a message to the world that we are in control? Or are we so frightened by the myriad possibilities and dangers before us that we attempt to retreat from this simultaneously thrilling and dangerous world of opportunity—even from adulthood itself—with our all-absorbing food obsessions and our Peter Pan bodies?

It is significant that eating disorders typically strike during the teenage and college years, at the times when we are forming our own identities and preparing to leave our families and define ourselves as independent beings. Other cultures have rites of passage, marking and celebrating the transition between childhood and womanhood. It is telling that so many young Western women, in contrast, fear this transition so much that they mark it by beginning a lifelong cycle of dieting, bingeing, and starving.

It may be that the roots of food preoccupation and obsessive dieting are different for each of us. But every one of us trapped by food preoccupation—whether we are typical dieters, anorexics, or bulimics—is, in effect, validating what Kim Chernin calls our culture's "tyranny of slenderness." And, as we grow into adulthood and raise our own children, we are perpetrating this tyranny and inflicting it on a new generation of women. As men, too, increasingly become victims of body stereotypes, our sons as well as our daughters are in danger.

Breaking the Cycle

Tyranny, however, can be stopped. You can define beauty as what's *normal and healthy* for your body. You can take off excess weight without agreeing to starvation diets that eat away at your muscles and bones. You can exercise to make your body fit and shapely rather than to strip it down to skin and bones. And you can recognize that you may be a natural size 2 or a natural size 12—and be happy at whichever is the perfect, healthy size for you.

When you do so, you'll free yourself to have a healthy, attractive, normal body, not a sick, sad body that puts you at risk for brittle bones, heart disease, depression, and deadly eating disorders. The power to recognize and reject dangerous cultural stereotypes, and the effect that these stereotypes have on your relationship with food and your body, is yours—and making the right choice will open the door to permanent weight loss and the beautiful body you deserve.

Some Food for Thought

- The typical "quick weight loss" diet in America restricts caloric intake to around nine hundred calories per day. The starvation diet fed to prisoners in Nazi concentration camps during World War II was eight to nine hundred calories per day.[23]

(continued)

• A recent study found that *Playboy* playmates have a body mass low enough to be considered unhealthy. "Given the perception of *Playboy* centerfolds as culturally ideal women," the researchers say, "the notion that 70 percent of them are underweight highlights the social pressure on women to be thin."[24]

• The average American woman is 5'4" and weighs 144 pounds. The average model is 5'9" and weighs 123 pounds.

• Gymnast Christy Henrich, who stood 4'10" and weighed 93 pounds, was a contender for an Olympic medal when she overheard a judge say, "She's too fat to make the Olympic gymnastic team." When she died from anorexia nervosa two years later, Henrich weighed 47 pounds.

• If Barbie were a real woman, she'd have to walk on all fours. She's too top-heavy to stand upright.

• A recent study in the *Journal of the American Medical Association* reported that in the 1920s Miss America contestants had body mass indexes well within the range considered healthy. Since that time, the researchers found, the average weight of pageant contestants has decreased by 12 percent, "putting an increasing number of winners in the range of under-nutrition."[25]

• A Stanford study found that 68 percent of college students felt worse about their own looks after reading women's magazines. Another study found that subjects viewing slides of thin models felt worse about themselves than subjects viewing slides of average or large models.

• If shop mannequins were real women, they'd be too thin to menstruate.

Part II

Steps One Through Three

*Do Your Homework to Prepare
Yourself for Diet-Free Weight Loss*

ARE YOU READY to break free from the prison of dieting or overeating?

The ten steps will teach you to take control of your eating, lose excess pounds, and maintain your ideal weight—without dieting and without sacrificing your own needs—for the rest of your life.

In Steps One through Three, I ask you to direct your focus toward yourself, becoming aware of your beliefs about food and your body and how these beliefs are influenced by our culture. Gaining this insight is the critical first stage of change, which will help free you from the barriers that lock you into a tense and uneasy relationship with food and your body and cause unnecessary weight gain.

Step One: Recognize Your Exhaustion

Test Yourself—Is Food Preoccupation Running Your Life?

"In the final analysis, dieting is a thief. It robs you of your time, your energy, your health, your money and your well-being."

Health writer Raena Morgan[1]

IF YOU'RE READING this book, it's because you've tried, time after time, to control your weight through dieting. Perhaps you spent a fortune on diet books or joined Jenny Craig or Weight Watchers, but couldn't control your weight. Maybe you tried the Atkins diet, the cabbage diet, the Sugar Busters Diet, the Carbohydrate Lover's Diet, and Dean Ornish's diet, and you still struggle with extra pounds. Or perhaps you've given up on the hope of ever being thin, unwilling to forfeit the pleasure of food for a sexy body and believing that you can't have both.

If so, you're tired of your life being reduced to what you ate for dinner or how much your body weighs on a scale. You're tired of disliking your body and not being able to change it. You're exhausted with saying to yourself, "I need to lose twenty pounds before my sister's wedding/my vacation/my graduation." You're tired of avoiding, craving, and fearing food or of overeating and suffering the consequences. In short, you're **Fed Up.**

If dieting is becoming an overwhelming force in your life, you may be scared that you'll keep gaining weight, that you won't be able to stop bingeing, or that your dieting is destroying your health and wasting your life. And if you've rebelled against endless dieting and resigned yourself to being trapped in an overweight body, you find yourself exhausted by the effort of being a "plus size" in a world that isn't kind to large people.

Does any of this sound familiar? If so, the first step in overcoming your fears and escaping from endless and unsuccessful dieting (or its counterpart, compulsive overeating) is to come to terms with how much your concerns about your weight and body size are affecting your life. Many people who complete this questionnaire—including people who consider themselves perfectly "normal" dieters, and people who've given up dieting and say they've come to terms with being overweight—are surprised to realize just how all-consuming their focus on weight and food has become. Armed with the self-awareness you'll gain from this questionnaire, you'll be ready to take steps to free yourself from the energy-sapping, esteem-lowering, fruitless merry-go-round of dieting and overeating—and ready to learn how to become fit, healthy, and attractive for life, while having a relaxed and even fun relationship with food. (Yes—it *is* possible to enjoy food and still have an attractive body!)

I hope you're ready to take your first steps away from unproductive, maladaptive dieting, or the compulsive overeating that often follows years of failed diets, and toward a fit and healthy body and a relaxed relationship with food. If you are, my Ten-Step No-Diet Fitness Plan will lead you to a freer, happier, fitter, and more meaningful life.

To start, you'll need two simple tools: courage and a pencil.

Why the pencil? Because the first step toward freeing yourself from a prison is to recognize that you're trapped. That's why I'm asking you to take a little time to complete the following questionnaire, which is designed to help you identify your own weight and food preoccupations and come to grips with the extent to which they control your life.

And why will you need courage? Because I know, as a former dieter, that the hardest lock to break on the door of the prison of dieting is the lock labeled *fear*. For years I was terrified to give up dieting and calorie counting, because I believed I would lose control of my eating and my weight. It takes a great leap of faith to believe that you can and should stop dieting if you want to get control of your weight, but if you're at the point where you realize that dieting doesn't work, you're ready to make that leap. You're ready to learn that dieting is what puts pounds on and that it's possible to eat what you want, when you want, and be attractive, happy, and in control of your body and appetite.

What do you have to gain? If you're a repetitive dieter, you'll gain a healthy and attractive body and freedom from endless diets that don't work and that actually increase your weight and endanger your health. If you've given up on dieting and resigned yourself to being overweight, you'll gain the tools you need to win the figure you thought wasn't possible, while still eating the foods you enjoy. And when you put down the burden of food and body preoccupation, you'll gain the freedom to be beautiful, fit, and "at home" with your body, without paying the unnecessary price of hunger, guilt, and self-denial.

What do you have to lose? The feeling of self-disgust when you step on the scales after a binge or a failed diet and see the numbers go up. The deprivation you feel when you turn down a party invitation because you're unhappy with your appearance or fear that you'll "pig out." The unending treadmill of calorie counting, food restriction, and self-punishing exercise, none of which has helped you achieve permanent weight loss and self-acceptance. The humiliation of overeating and feeling helpless and "out of control."

If you think you're ready to make this change, take the first step by completing the simple fifty-item "Are You Exhausted?" self-inventory that follows. I recommend finding a quiet and restful place, where you feel calm and relaxed and can think about the questions carefully as you answer them. Some people feel self-conscious completing a questionnaire like this, but remember that when it comes to your health and your life, *what you know can never hurt you as much as what you don't know.*

Participating in this questionnaire may cause you some anxiety or even anger, because looking honestly at maladaptive behavior patterns can be an uncomfortable experience. But self-awareness is a necessary part of change, and change—while it can be frightening—is also the positive alternative to life patterns leading you away from, not toward, the body you deserve.

So take a deep breath, relax, and get started. Some tips on scoring yourself accurately:

- If you find it hard to choose between "yes" and "no," choose "yes" if you feel the question describes you more often than not.
- Think about the answers that best describe where you are now, today, unless you find that there are wide fluctuations in your scores over the past month. In that case, choose "yes" if the question describes you most of the time during the past month.
- Remember, most of the time means more than half of the time.

"Are You Exhausted?" Self-Inventory

Answer the following questions with a "yes" or "no" response. Choose "yes" if the question sounds like you most of the time.

1. Do you buy clothes that are too small for you because you plan to wear them later on when you're thinner?   ☐ Yes ☐ No

2. Do you diet in preparation for special events?   ☐ Yes ☐ No

3. Do you generally weigh yourself on a daily basis or even more often?   ☐ Yes ☐ No

4. Have you been on two or more diets in the past year, without achieving or maintaining the results you hoped for?   ☐ Yes ☐ No

5. Do you take a calorie inventory of all the foods you eat?   ☐ Yes ☐ No

6. Do you avoid or postpone certain activities because of concerns about your body?   ☐ Yes ☐ No

7. Do you avoid sexual activity, or attempt to keep your body hidden during sexual activity, because of concerns about your body?   ☐ Yes ☐ No

8. Do you wear baggy clothes because of concerns about your body size?   ☐ Yes ☐ No

9. Do you refuse to allow certain types of food in your home (for instance, ice cream) out of fear that you will binge? ☐ Yes ☐ No

10. Do you own several sizes of clothing because of weight fluctuations related to dieting? ☐ Yes ☐ No

11. Have you ever had medical problems because of the effects of dieting, weight cycling, or obesity? ☐ Yes ☐ No

12. Have you experienced irregular menstrual periods because of your eating and/or exercise patterns? ☐ Yes ☐ No

13. Do you feel physically uncomfortable or lethargic because of your weight? ☐ Yes ☐ No

14. Do you eat certain foods only after rationalizing that you will "make up" for it in some way? ☐ Yes ☐ No

15. Do you exercise to compensate for eating certain foods? ☐ Yes ☐ No

16. Do you ever pre-plan what you will eat when you go to parties or other social events? ☐ Yes ☐ No

17. Do you purge, or take laxatives, enemas, or diuretics to compensate for having eaten or in an attempt to control your weight? ☐ Yes ☐ No

18. Do you eat at specified times during the day or place restrictions on when you can eat? ☐ Yes ☐ No

19. Do you eat less when in public than you'd like to eat? ☐ Yes ☐ No

20. Do you eat in secret? ☐ Yes ☐ No

21. Do you feel that your moods fluctuate rapidly in relation to your food intake or your weight? ☐ Yes ☐ No

22. Do you feel out-of-control when you eat or fear eating
    because you are afraid you won't be able to stop?   ☐ Yes   ☐ No

23. Do you find that you frequently eat to the point where
    you feel bloated or sick?   ☐ Yes   ☐ No

24. Do you ever count how many bites of food you eat, or
    chew your food and then spit it out without swallowing
    it, in an attempt to control your weight?   ☐ Yes   ☐ No

25. Do you dread certain social situations because of the
    appearance of your body?   ☐ Yes   ☐ No

26. Has a doctor or other health professional expressed
    concern about you being underweight?   ☐ Yes   ☐ No

27. Is your self-esteem dependent or based greatly upon
    your weight or body size?   ☐ Yes   ☐ No

28. Do you ever eat only one food type during the course
    of a day, in an effort to control your weight?   ☐ Yes   ☐ No

29. Has your weight fluctuated by more than fifteen
    pounds in one month because of the effects of dieting?   ☐ Yes   ☐ No

30. Are you critical or envious of other people's weight or
    body shape?   ☐ Yes   ☐ No

31. Have you ever joined a weight loss organization, such
    as Jenny Craig, Weight Watchers, or Overeaters Anony-
    mous, but either failed to lose weight or gained back
    any weight you lost?   ☐ Yes   ☐ No

32. Do you use appetite suppressants or other drugs, either
    prescribed or illicit, in an attempt to control how much
    you eat?   ☐ Yes   ☐ No

33. Do you dream about food?   ☐ Yes   ☐ No

34. Do you skip meals when you're hungry, in an attempt to control your weight? ☐ Yes ☐ No

35. Do you have a mental list of foods that are acceptable and foods that are unacceptable? ☐ Yes ☐ No

36. Do you eat more than you intended, or eat foods that you feel you "shouldn't eat," and then feel a strong sense of guilt afterward? ☐ Yes ☐ No

37. Do you turn to food when you feel anxious, emotional, lonely, bored, or frustrated? ☐ Yes ☐ No

38. Do you often "zone out" and eat when you're not hungry, without paying attention to what you're eating? ☐ Yes ☐ No

39. Do you ever eat very large amounts of food, eat much more rapidly than what is generally considered normal, or eat far past the point of being physically hungry? ☐ Yes ☐ No

40. Are you distressed because of binge eating? ☐ Yes ☐ No

41. Do you feel depressed or ashamed about your weight, shape, and appearance? ☐ Yes ☐ No

42. Do you think about your food intake or your body size every day? ☐ Yes ☐ No

43. Do you greatly dislike your body and consider taking extreme measures to change it? ☐ Yes ☐ No

44. Do you attempt to pre-plan what you will allow yourself to eat at a meal, or find yourself feeling apprehensive or anxious before you sit down to a meal? ☐ Yes ☐ No

45. Do you feel that your body has to be perfect in order for you to be satisfied in life? ☐ Yes ☐ No

46. Have you had cosmetic surgery to change your body
    shape/size and later gained back the weight lost during
    the surgery?   ☐ Yes   ☐ No

47. When you drink beverages, do you choose exclusively
    water, beverages sweetened with sugar substitutes, or
    other low-calorie beverages (coffee, tea, etc.)?   ☐ Yes   ☐ No

48. Do you always seem to be trying to lose weight?   ☐ Yes   ☐ No

49. Do you feel a sense of a rush, or a sense of being dis-
    connected from the world and its problems, during a
    bingeing episode?   ☐ Yes   ☐ No

50. Do you feel your body size or weight is limiting your
    ability to enjoy your life?   ☐ Yes   ☐ No

Scoring

If you answered "yes" to any of the following questions, give yourself
  one point for each: 1, 2, 30, 37, 48
If you answered "yes" to any of the following questions, give yourself
  two points for each: 3, 4, 5, 8, 9, 10, 14, 15, 16, 18, 19, 33, 34, 35,
  36, 38, 39, 47
If you answered "yes" to any of the following questions, give yourself
  three points for each: 6, 13, 20, 21, 22, 23, 24, 25, 27, 28, 29, 31,
  32, 40, 41, 42, 43, 44, 45, 49, 50
If you answered "yes" to any of the following questions, give yourself
  four points for each: 7, 11, 12, 17, 26, 46

Note: Answering "yes" to any of the four-point questions or to a significant
number of other questions on this questionnaire may indicate that you are in need
of professional help beyond the scope of this book. If you have a serious problem
with eating and dieting, you could be at risk for medical and mental health disorders. Anorexia nervosa and bulimia nervosa are potentially life-threatening conditions, and dieting in and of itself can be dangerous. It's always best to be on the

safe side and pursue professional counseling and/or medical care if you have concerns about your preoccupations with dieting.

When you've finished scoring your answers, add up your total points.

0–20: You exhibit few signs of food and body preoccupations. You may experience distress and concern about your weight and shape, but overall you have effective strategies for dealing with your concerns. My Ten-Step No-Diet Fitness Plan can reinforce these strategies and offer you new techniques to achieve and maintain long-term weight loss. These steps will teach you how to be fit and attractive without developing dangerous food and body preoccupations and without dieting.

21–45: You exhibit evidence of food and body preoccupations significant enough to affect your self-esteem and place some limits on your life. You have some effective strategies but are probably still struggling with unsuccessful dieting. Your strategies are not always positive, and they may take a significant toll on your mental and physical energy. If so, the Ten-Step No-Diet Fitness Plan can help you learn better, more enduring, and more effective ways to achieve healthy weight and fitness goals.

46–70: You spend a great deal of your time worrying about food and body concerns, and your concerns are taking a significant toll on your mental and physical energy and well-being. You have a tense and uncomfortable relationship with food or your body, and your concerns probably manifest in other areas of your life, limiting your ability to live in the present and be satisfied with your life. Are you ready to challenge the belief system that has failed to provide you with the body you desire? If so, my Ten-Step No-Diet Fitness Plan will help you develop a more effective, stress-free, and long-lasting approach to weight loss, health, and fitness.

71–95: Food and body concerns are a very significant stressor, causing you a great deal of emotional pain. Turning to one diet after another has taken a significant toll on your self-esteem. Your concerns are very likely to affect many areas of your life, and your dissatisfaction with your body may impede your ability to form or enjoy intimate relationships. You're caught up in the vicious cycle of dieting unsuccessfully and limiting your ability to enjoy food and your life. The Ten-Step No-Diet Fitness Plan can help you achieve permanent weight loss and transform your nerve-racking relationship with food and your body into a relaxed and satisfied relationship.

96 and up: Food and body concerns dominate your day-to-day routine. Others may not know it, and even you yourself may not be aware of the degree to which repetitive dieting has overtaken your life, but you are probably in a great deal of emotional pain. Your social life and health are likely to be limited severely because of your approach to weight management. Dieting and concerns about your weight are most likely severely affecting your self-esteem and causing you guilt and mental anguish. It's crucial that you make a change, for the sake of your emotional well-being and physical health. The Ten-Step No-Diet Fitness Plan can offer you new hope and show you how to break free from unsuccessful and destructive dieting patterns, lose your excess pounds, and attain a healthy, sexy, attractive body. It will take courage to do this, but remember: *dieting hasn't worked for you,* so you have nothing to lose and the rest of your life to gain.

Armed with the insight you've gained from this questionnaire, you're ready to become fit and diet-free. No matter how many years you've sacrificed, and how many failed diets you've endured, you can break free of your self-destructive pattern of dieting, bingeing, or overeating. If you're ready to let go of the burden of dieting and discover a successful diet-free path to fitness, you're ready for the Ten-Step No-Diet Fitness Plan program.

It's time to recognize that despite the pain and self-sacrifice you've endured in hopes of achieving a healthy body through dieting, you haven't been able to control your weight. It's time to believe that you can have a natural and relaxed relationship with food and also have a sexy and healthy body. It's time to take back your life . . . starting now. It's time to get **Fed Up!**

Step Two: Reject the Cultural Myths That Make You Diet and *Gain* Weight

"A survey found just one percent of young women are completely happy with the shape of their body [and that] one in ten have taken drugs to try and achieve their ideal weight. . . . Seventy percent felt depressed about their shape or size. . . . One in ten had suffered from anorexia, 9% had suffered bulimia, and 21% admitted they had binged on food."

BBC News, February 21, 2001[1]

"Many males are becoming insecure about their physical appearance as advertising and other media images raise the standard and idealize well-built men. Researchers [are seeing] an alarming increase in obsessive weight training and the use of anabolic steroids and dietary supplements that promise bigger muscles or more stamina for lifting."

Body Image and Advertising, Issue Briefs, 2000[2]

IN CHAPTER 3 I talked about our culture's dangerous myths about body image. In this step I want you to think hard about *what these myths do to you personally*—and then I want you to find, within yourself, the strength to reject them.

Why? Because to be truly fit and attractive, and lose your excess weight permanently, you need to do what's right for you and your body. But modern Western culture actually teaches you that attractiveness depends on denigrating and harming yourself. If you surrender to this ideology, it will damage your health, crush your spirit, limit your life, and drive you even farther away from having the beautiful body you deserve. Reject your culture's dangerous message, however, and you will be free to follow your individual path to health, fitness, and beauty.

The first step in becoming fit and diet-free is to recognize the tyranny of our modern "anorexic culture" and release yourself from it. That doesn't mean that you can't be beautiful and healthy. *You can!* If you are overweight, you can lose excess pounds. If you are out of shape, you can become fit and firm. You can have a body that will look fabulous in an evening gown, a tuxedo, or a swimsuit.

To attain a beautiful and healthy body, however, *you must define beautiful and healthy in a realistic way*. Otherwise you'll forever be chasing a brass ring that can't be caught, and you'll spend your life trapped in dieting and weight cycling. The result, as I explained in Chapter 2: you'll gain weight, not lose it.

Thus, before you take *physical* steps to change your life and lose your excess weight, it's critical to take some *mental* steps. The first and most important is to get rid of the cultural baggage that's holding you back from being attractive, healthy, and happy.

Conduct a "Media Watch"

To gain insight into the flood of cultural images influencing your ideas about beauty—and, in particular, about how much you should weigh to be attractive—I want you to conduct a small research project. For a single day, from the time you get up until you go to bed, pay attention to all of the messages about weight that you receive from advertisers and the media (television, movies, radio, books, magazines, newspapers).

For instance:

- Watch the news shows. Do you see any females whose figures you would consider typical?
- Watch television soap operas, sitcoms, drama shows, or TV movies. Do you see any women larger than a size 6 or any men over about 180 pounds? If so, are they romantic leads or "character" actors (e.g., comic sidekicks)?
- If you watch a movie, do any of the romantic characters, male or female, weigh as much as you and your friends? In contrast, do the character actors look like the average people you know?
- Leaf through the books you're reading. How are the main characters' bodies described? Are any of the romantic interests an average size or "full figured," or are they all slender?
- In the grocery line, scan the covers of the magazines on the racks. Do any of them have photos of average-sized male models or female models who weigh more than 120 pounds?
- Look at the billboards as you drive. Do you see anyone who *isn't* abnormally thin advertising any product pertaining to health or beauty? Do you see anyone who isn't thin advertising glamorous products such as sports cars?
- Look at product brochures, college catalogs, cookbooks, even how-to manuals. Do they include any photos of women over a size 8 or of large men?
- Watch music videos on MTV or VH1. Do you see any men or women who look like the people you know?
- Leaf through clothing catalogs. What percentage of the models are the same sizes and shapes as the real-life men and women buying the clothing they advertise?

By the end of the day, you'll have viewed several hundred images on TV, in magazines, or in videos—and almost all of those images will be of men and women far thinner than an average, healthy size. Your "media watch" will open your eyes to the amount of propaganda you internalize every day. If you're a woman, this propaganda tells you that you're not attractive unless you weigh less than 97 percent of American females. If you're a man, it tells you that sexy men must have slender, V-shaped bodies or the type of muscles that can be achieved only by constantly working out (or taking steroids). In short, *you're taught that you MUST achieve a look that statistics say you CAN'T achieve naturally*—a recipe for disappointment, "diet fatigue," and heartbreak.

> *Claudia, a woman I met recently, immigrated to the United States about four years ago from Guatemala. In her own country she never thought about her weight. In fact, because she's short and thinner than many of the women in her country, she thought of herself as petite.*
>
> *After a few months of being in the states, Claudia began to compare her body to the bodies of the models and actresses who exemplify America's "ideal" look and to feel ungainly and unattractive. She gave up her favorite McDonald's combo lunch and began her first diet, and then a second, and then a third. Before long, she switched to diet pills, which temporarily took off weight but made her nauseated and anxious.*
>
> *The result of Claudia's efforts, not surprisingly, is that she's gained twenty pounds. Worse, in the process she's lost her easy confidence and her belief in her own beauty. She tells me now, "I feel disgusted with myself." She's planning on starting another diet, even though the salad-all-day diet, the temporary fast, and the low-carb diet didn't work.*
>
> *How did American culture change Claudia? Five years ago she looked in the mirror and liked the petite woman looking back. Today she starves herself to the point of weakness—and yet when she looks in the mirror, she sees a "fat" woman, gross and unacceptable. And when I look at Claudia, I see an eating disorder, or a lifetime of diet-caused weight gain, in the making.*

Claudia wasn't overweight when she arrived in the United States, yet just a few months in our media-saturated culture convinced her that she looked "fat" and "ugly." Imagine how hard life is for women who *do* need to trim down to reach a healthy weight! They're told that they must diet not to a normal weight but to abnormal thinness, and yet every diet they try puts pounds on rather than taking them off. It's a battle that can't be won by anyone—except the diet industry.

Take a Close Look at Diet Claims and Diet Reality

Part of the cultural "pollution" you swim in each day is the astounding number of newspaper, magazine, and TV ads for diets and diet products.

You know the ones I'm talking about. There are the ads that say "Jane's ex-husband is sorry he divorced her now that she's a size 6!" There are the ads for the book *Suzanne Somers' Get Skinny on Fabulous Food*—as though skinniness and gauntness, rather than an attractive, sexy, curved body, should be the goal. And there's *Body for Life*, in which Bill Phillips shows "before" pictures (some of people who aren't overweight to begin with) and "after" pictures of people who lost weight after twelve weeks on his diet, but admits that he put up cash prizes and his "blood-red Lamborghini Diablo" as rewards to entice these dieters to lose weight. (Not surprisingly, he also adds the disclaimer, "They achieved extraordinary results; there are no typical results.")

The diet industry willingly colludes in the media's effort to make you feel inadequate and ugly if you can't diet your way to an inhumanly perfect body, and the reason is obvious. Virtually anyone can achieve an attractive, healthy weight, but it's nearly impossible for the majority of us to look like Brad Pitt or Jennifer Aniston. And diet gurus love impossible goals! To them a customer who buys four diet books and hundreds of dollars' worth of diet foods and pills each year, and never loses weight in the long run, is a dream customer. Thus they're happy when you make it your goal to become impossibly thin and then fail at that goal, over and over and over again.

Some men and women see through this game and stop dieting—but by then diets have robbed many of them of the ability to eat naturally, leading them to become overeaters who believe that they are helplessly out of control. Others continue, year after year, to fulfill the diet industry's fantasies, while crushing their own dreams with endless diets that leave them discouraged, tired, and more overweight than before.

You can continue to be the diet industry's dream customer or to kick yourself for being "weak" if you've given up on dieting—or you can recognize the fact that miracle diets haven't worked and never will. To make this choice, it helps to fully understand the futility of your past or current dieting efforts. This simple activity will help you:

Truth in Dieting Analysis

1. Take several sheets of paper. At the top of each sheet, list the name of a diet you've tried. This should include *any plan that imposes limits on what you can eat.* (For instance, Dean Ornish's book *Eat More, Weigh Less* contains a section on what you should and shouldn't eat, making it a diet plan.) On additional sheets of paper, list diet pills or diet foods you've used.

2. On each sheet, list your recollections of how you felt before beginning the diet or using the diet product. Did you buy a book promoting the diet? Did the book list many impressive-sounding scientific reasons why the diet would work? (For instance, did it promise that the combination of foods it allowed contained special chemicals that would "melt off" your fat or say that you would lose weight by putting your body in a state of ketosis?) Did the pills or diet foods promise miracle results in a convincing way?

3. Describe how you felt when you began each diet or started using each diet product. Were you hopeful, excited, optimistic?

4. Describe what happened during the first few weeks that you dieted or used the diet product. Did you lose weight quickly? Did you enjoy the compliments of friends and family? Did you believe that the diet would solve your weight problems—perhaps all of your problems—for good?

5. Describe what happened as you continued to diet or use the diet pills or foods. Did the diet or diet product continue to work, and did you lose the weight you had hoped to lose and keep it off? Or did you regain the weight and possibly even more? If so, how did you feel, physically and emotionally, when your diet failed?

6. Now look at your list and make several estimates. First, calculate how much time you invested in each diet or diet product and how much weight you lost *over the long term* as a result. Second, calculate the amount of money you spent on each diet or diet product. In addition, note the emotional effects of each diet you tried.

If you're a typical "serial dieter," your results will show that you've invested a tremendous amount of time and hundreds if not thousands of dollars for no long-term benefit at all. In fact you probably weigh more now than you did when you first decided to lose weight! In addition, your list will reveal the high emotional price of the diets that failed you. Typical postdiet emotions that dieters list in point 5 are "sadness," "tiredness," "a sense of failure," "a feeling of hopelessness," and "self-loathing"—a poor reward for weeks or months of deprivation.

What does this mean? It means that unnatural cultural expectations have suckered you into becoming a perpetual dieter and that the diet industry is benefiting by taking you for hundreds (or possibly thousands) of dollars—while you wind up feeling overweight, ugly, and defeated. You're a victim of a one-two whammy: a society that holds up impossible images of beauty and a profit-crazed industry that uses those images to sell you modern-day snake oil.

Acknowledge the Inner Toll of Dieting

The financial damage caused by your endless pursuit of the "perfect" body is obvious. In addition, there is the physical damage: when you diet, you feel weak and hungry, and you deprive your body of the fuel and nutrients it needs. When you stop dieting, you regain the weight and usually more. And yo-yo dieting, as I explained in Chapter 2, damages your bones, your heart, and your overall health.

But the psychological toll of perpetual dieting is equally great, if not greater. As a psychotherapist, I work with many "serial dieters." Some are young, many still in their teens or twenties. Yet they seem older than their years, their sparkle and self-confidence replaced by anxiety and weariness. Others come to me in their forties or fifties, perplexed and dissatisfied after dieting for decades and continuing to gain weight. The faces and posture of these special, wonderful, yet suffering women and men show the strain and weariness of soldiers fighting an endless losing battle.

After losing more than a decade of my life to the same battle, one thing I remember clearly is being incredibly tired. At twelve I felt smart and pretty, bursting with energy, and optimistic about my future. At twenty-two I felt tired, defeated, inadequate, and ugly. I knew that dieting and the pursuit of narrow and artificial beauty goals controlled my life, but I couldn't stop until I recognized the true enemy.

That enemy—the same one that traps you in the cycle of dieting and overeating and keeps you from achieving true health and fitness—is a culture that tells you "Normal isn't good enough." Dieting exhausts you, because it demands the impossible: that you diet and exercise your body into a size and shape that *can't be attained* by 97 percent of men or women.

If this struggle wears you down to the point where you say "Enough!" and give up on the goal of having a healthy and sexy body, you'll be left with excess pounds and the feeling that you will never be able to control your eating or your weight. Worse yet, you'll feel tremendous unwarranted guilt over your "failure," because you won't recognize that it was the diets that failed and not you.

Conversely, if you continue to try diet after diet, the psychological toll will be just as high. If you're a serial dieter, it's important to recognize the degree to which repetitive dieting affects your life, saps your energy, and steals your optimism and enthusiasm for life. Ask yourself:

- Do you wake up eager and happy most mornings—or do you almost immediately begin worrying about your weight and/or what you'll eat during the day?
- Are holidays, weddings, birthdays, and other food-filled get-togethers fun for you? Or do you wear yourself out worrying about how you'll look, what you can wear to look "less fat," and what you can and can't eat?
- Do you often feel weak and hungry but refuse to eat because your diet won't let you?
- Do you often go for days or weeks eating too little food to keep your body functioning well?
- Do you exercise even when you don't want to, or even when you don't feel good, because you "have to"?
- Do you spend a large part of your time and energy each day worrying about your weight and comparing yourself to men or women who you think are more attractive?
- When you think about your future, do you find yourself weighed down by the thought of endless dieting and the fear that you'll never be able to reach and maintain an attractive weight?
- Do you believe that you'll never be "good enough," no matter what you achieve, unless you are thin?
- Does your dieting exhaust the people around you? If you're a parent, do your children have to live with your "high" each time you start a new diet and your "low" each time it fails? Are they forced to accept

odd and ever-changing menu plans and to tolerate your irritability when you're hungry or your weight plateaus? Does your spouse or partner find it hard to cope with your mood swings, your weight yo-yoing, and the "I can't" syndrome ("Thanks for the chocolates, but I can't eat them"; "Yes, it looks like a fun restaurant, but I can't get anything 'legal' there"; "I know you want to go to the reunion, but I can't let them see me like this")?

If you answered yes to many of these questions, it may be time to recognize the full price that you and your loved ones are paying for your failed diets—a price that includes stunted dreams and goals, low self-esteem, anger, frustration, and damage to both your body and your psyche. And realize that you will continue to pay this price, over and over, until you gain the strength to reject corrupt cultural standards and break free from the prison of endless dieting.

Define Your Own Beauty

Western culture teaches you that you must re-create yourself as an anorexic goddess or an impossibly sculpted god. The diet industry, in turn, tells you that dieting will make your body perfect and that you are to blame when dieting fails. Thus you become trapped in a cycle of starving and bingeing while your physical and mental health suffers and your loved ones suffer along with you.

To break this cycle, and achieve true fitness and attractiveness, you must begin by answering a simple question: what weight is right for you?

Don't let the simplicity of this question fool you, because to answer it you need to reject years of cultural conditioning. That conditioning is every bit as powerful as the social attitudes that once made many African-Americans feel that they were ugly simply because they weren't white. And it's every bit as powerful as the cultural brainwashing that made women in the mid-1800s lace themselves into corsets so tight that they damaged their internal organs, deformed their spines, and sometimes even crushed their unborn babies to death.

Like people in these eras, we find it hard to see the toxic effects of our culture. But like the early feminists who refused to corset their waists, or the African-Americans who led the "Black Is Beautiful" movement of the 1960s, we must take back our bodies from the people who would weaken or even kill us to make a profit.

If you accept this challenge, the next step is to define your own standard of healthy beauty. If you shouldn't strive to look like Kate Moss, whom should you look like? The answer is simple: you should look like yourself—at the weight that's the most healthy and attractive for *you*. But how, after years of conditioning, can you even know what your body should look like?

You can't create an exact picture of your ideal body, but you can make a realistic estimate of your proper weight. That weight has nothing to do with the weight of the cover models in *GQ* or *Mademoiselle*. Instead it has to do with reality: the reality of your genetic heritage, your age, your fitness level, and your medical status.

To gain insight into what weight range is attractive and healthy for you, consider the following factors.

Your Genes

Wouldn't it be great if we could mold our bodies like Play-Doh? We'd simply squeeze out bigger boobs, flatten our butts, or restructure our pecs, depending on what our country and our times demanded. But we're not made of modeling clay. We're made of flesh and bone and built according to a blueprint designed by our genes—and those genes don't care what's "in" or "out."

Dozens of these genes regulate how easy it is for you to put on weight and how hard it is for you to take it off. To get a feel for your genetic blueprint, look at your family members. If many are tall, the odds are you're tall, too. If many are "busty," you're probably endowed with genes that dictate a large bust size. If many are pear shaped or apple shaped, you may be genetically predisposed to put on weight in the same places. And if most of your family members gain weight easily and lose it slowly, you're probably endowed with genes that hoard fat efficiently.

That *doesn't* mean that you're doomed to be overweight if your relatives are, because both genetic and environmental factors play a role in how prone you are to weight gain. But your genes will definitely influence whether you're naturally lithe, lanky, voluptuous, curvy, broad shouldered or small chested. It's a fact of life—and trying to circumvent it will set you up for failure.

Michelle wasn't overweight, but she started dieting in her teens, shortly after she lost the leading role in her high school's production of Romeo and Juliet *to a thinner girl. "I blamed it on my big hips," she says, "because the girl who won the role was tiny." Adopting a grueling and rigid eating plan that entailed fasting every other day and eating only very low-fat foods, Michelle lost twenty-five pounds—far more than she should have, leaving her face and arms gaunt—but she continued to be obsessed by her wide hips, which she still couldn't fit into the tiny size-6 jeans she coveted.*

Finally, a friend gave Michelle a reality check. "I hadn't seen him in two years," she says, "and when I opened the door he immediately said, 'What's the matter—are you sick?' At that point I started to wonder what I was doing to myself." Another turning point came at a family reunion, when Michelle looked around her and realized that none of the women in her family, no matter what their weight, had the tiny hips and buttocks she was striving to attain. "It dawned on me," she says, "that if I starved myself to death, I'd go to my grave with size-10 hips." It took additional time for Michelle to come to terms with the knowledge that she's a natural size 10 and not a natural size 6—but she's healthier, and looks far more sexy and attractive, now that she's no longer trying to be someone she isn't.

Your Age

As we grow older, most of us put on weight more easily and have more difficulty taking it off. Thus, even if you were a size 8 when you graduated from college, you may be a natural size 10 or 12 in your forties—and if you're a man whose wedding suit had a size-30 waist, don't be surprised if you're naturally a 31 or 32 when you reach midlife. Once you enter your twenties, your body generally begins losing a small amount of muscle mass each year, even if you get plenty of exercise. This causes your metabolic rate to slow down, which means that you get more "mileage" from the calories that you eat—and that, in turn, means that you'll naturally add a few pounds in your thirties and forties. This isn't abnormal or unhealthy. Again, it's just a fact of life, and it means that you may need to adjust your mental image of your ideal body as you age.

Your Hormones

Leptin, a hormone that helps control appetite and reduce the body's ability to store fat, is currently the object of much scientific interest. But it's only one of a symphony of hormones that affect how our bodies handle food. Because of our genetic diversity, we have different levels of these chemicals and differing abilities to gain or lose weight.

For women, reproductive hormones also play a role in weight control. Women frequently put on a few pounds at menopause, when hormonal changes tend to make them add weight around their waists. Women also tend to gain weight after each pregnancy, and it takes time for that weight to come off. It's important for women at these stages of life to be realistic about their weight and about the fact that taking off any excess pounds will require patience.

Medical Conditions

In Chapter 9 I talk about the importance of identifying any medical conditions that affect your weight. It's also important to take these medical issues into account when setting your fitness goals. If you're at risk for developing diabetes, for instance, losing a significant amount of weight may be vital to your long-term health. If you have polycystic ovarian disease, you'll need to recognize that the disorder makes weight loss more difficult. If you're sedentary because of illness or injury, you'll need to set weight goals that you can realistically achieve with a minimum of activity. In short, your health profile will dictate, at least to some degree, both how much weight you should lose and how long it may take you to lose it.

Your "Settling Point"

In Chapter 2 I discussed the concept of a "settling point"—the weight at which your body naturally tends to stay if you are not starving yourself or overeating. Your body will tend to return to this weight when you stop dieting and start eating naturally. But remember that your "settling point" is a factor of *both genes and environment* and isn't set in stone. If you previously were a couch potato and ate only high-fat foods, your "settling point" will most likely be significantly lower if you exercise and eventually begin eating a good variety of foods.

Body Mass Index Chart

Body Weight (pounds)

BMI / Height (inches)	19	20	21	22	23	24	25	26	27	28	29	30	31	32	33	34	35	36	37	38	39	40	41	42	43	44	45	46	47	48	49	50	51	52	53	54
58	91	96	100	105	110	115	119	124	129	134	138	143	148	153	158	162	167	172	177	181	186	191	196	201	205	210	215	220	224	229	234	239	244	248	253	258
59	94	99	104	109	114	119	124	128	133	138	143	148	153	158	163	168	173	178	183	188	193	198	203	208	212	217	222	227	232	237	242	247	252	257	262	267
60	97	102	107	112	118	123	128	133	138	143	148	153	158	163	168	174	179	184	189	194	199	204	209	215	220	225	230	235	240	245	250	255	261	266	271	276
61	100	106	111	116	122	127	132	137	143	148	153	158	164	169	174	180	185	190	195	201	206	211	217	222	227	232	238	243	248	254	259	264	269	275	280	285
62	104	109	115	120	126	131	136	142	147	153	158	164	169	175	180	186	191	196	202	207	213	218	224	229	235	240	246	251	256	262	267	273	278	284	289	295
63	107	113	118	124	130	135	141	146	152	158	163	169	175	180	186	191	197	203	208	214	220	225	231	237	242	248	254	259	265	270	278	282	287	293	299	304
64	110	116	122	128	134	140	145	151	157	163	169	174	180	186	192	197	204	209	215	221	227	232	238	244	250	256	262	267	273	279	285	291	296	302	308	314
65	114	120	126	132	138	144	150	156	162	168	174	180	186	192	198	204	210	216	222	228	234	240	246	252	258	264	270	276	282	288	294	300	306	312	318	324
66	118	124	130	136	142	148	155	161	167	173	179	186	192	198	204	210	216	223	229	235	241	247	253	260	266	272	278	284	291	297	303	309	315	322	328	334
67	121	127	134	140	146	153	159	166	172	178	185	191	198	204	211	217	223	230	236	242	249	255	261	268	274	280	287	293	299	306	312	319	325	331	338	344
68	125	131	138	144	151	158	164	171	177	184	190	197	203	210	216	223	230	236	243	249	256	262	269	276	282	289	295	302	308	315	322	328	335	341	348	354
69	128	135	142	149	155	162	169	176	182	189	196	203	209	216	223	230	236	243	250	257	263	270	277	284	291	297	304	311	318	324	331	338	345	351	358	365
70	132	139	146	153	160	167	174	181	188	195	202	209	216	222	229	236	243	250	257	264	271	278	285	292	299	306	313	320	327	334	341	348	355	362	369	376
71	136	143	150	157	165	172	179	186	193	200	208	215	222	229	236	243	250	257	265	272	279	286	293	301	308	315	322	329	338	343	351	358	365	372	379	386
72	140	147	154	162	169	177	184	191	199	206	213	221	228	235	242	250	258	265	272	279	287	294	302	309	316	324	331	338	346	353	361	368	375	383	390	397
73	144	151	159	166	174	182	189	197	204	212	219	227	235	242	250	257	265	272	280	288	295	302	310	318	325	333	340	348	355	363	371	378	386	393	401	408
74	148	155	163	171	179	186	194	202	210	218	225	233	241	249	256	264	272	280	287	295	303	311	319	326	334	342	350	358	365	373	381	389	396	404	412	420
75	152	160	168	176	184	192	200	208	216	224	232	240	248	256	264	272	279	287	295	303	311	319	327	335	343	351	359	367	375	383	391	399	407	415	423	431
76	156	164	172	180	189	197	205	213	221	230	238	246	254	263	271	279	287	295	304	312	320	328	336	344	353	361	369	377	385	394	402	410	418	426	435	443

(Source: Adapted from Clinical Guidelines on the Identification, Evaluation, and Treatment of Overweight and Obesity in Adults: The Evidence Report.)

Your Realistic Body Mass

In general it's a good idea to throw away the charts and graphs that claim to tell you what your correct weight is. These charts are often unscientific or even bizarre. (A friend of mine still remembers one celebrity's formula for calculating an ideal weight—a formula that told my friend that, at 5′6″, she should weigh between 99 and 112 pounds. Yet at the low end of that "ideal" range, my friend would probably suffer many of the health effects associated with anorexia!)

However, you can get some idea of the weight range that's healthy for your body by calculating your body mass. You've probably heard of the "body mass index," or BMI, a somewhat more accurate system than weight charts. (I think of the BMI as the "least bad" of the systems for calculating a realistic weight goal.) On the preceding page is the body mass index currently used by government agencies.

You can also calculate your BMI by using this formula: Multiply your weight (in pounds) by 704.5; multiply your height (in inches) by your height (in inches). Divide the first result by the second. For example:

If you're 5′5″ (65 inches) and weigh 140:
 140 × 704.5 = 98630
 65 × 65 = 4225
 98630 ÷ 4225 = 23
Thus, your BMI is 23.

Here's how BMI scores are typically interpreted. However, many professionals consider these limits to be too strict and suggest that there is little evidence that a BMI between 25 and 30 is unhealthy. In one massive review of the research on weight and dieting, for instance, D. M. Garner and S. C. Wolley concluded that the adverse effects of being somewhat overweight "are in fact the subject of considerable controversy," noting that "examination of the actual mortality data from many epidemiological studies makes it clear that, across studies, there is often no reliable pattern of association between premature death and relative weight."[3]

Less than 18.5:	Underweight
18.5 to 24.9:	Healthy Weight
25.0 to 29.9:	Overweight

30.0 to 34.9:	Obese
35.0 to 39.9:	Significantly Obese
40.0 or higher:	Extremely Obese

BMI charts aren't valid if you're pregnant, nursing, elderly, or a highly competitive athlete, and they don't reflect the fact that there are significant differences between men and women. More important, while your BMI is a better guide than weight charts, it's at best a ballpark estimate. If you're healthy and attractive at a BMI of 29, or if you're naturally thin and your BMI is 17.5 even when you don't diet, don't obsess over the numbers.

The key fact to recognize, in looking at the BMI chart, is there's a *very wide range* in "healthy" weight. (For example, a weight range of 120 to 158 pounds is considered healthy for a person who is 5′7″.) That's because nature loves diversity, and thus we have dozens (possibly even hundreds) of genes that play a role in varying our heights and weights.

That *doesn't* mean, however, that you're meant to be overweight or obese. In reality, very few of us are genetically wired for obesity. If you're over-weight right now, you can gradually lose excess weight and keep it off when your body recovers from the unnatural starvation mode that dieting forced on it. But the fact that we come in a variety of shapes means that you're probably not meant to be a size 6.

I thought about this fact the other night while my husband and I were watching a WNBA game. The women who play professional basketball are as fit as it's possible to be and are among the most elite of women athletes. They get hours of strenuous exercise almost every day; many have personal trainers or even personal chefs. If there were one "perfect" body size, they'd all have it! But the stats show otherwise. Four of the players on the court that night were 5′9″, but one weighed 130, another 162, and the others 148 and 150. That's a 32-pound weight difference between these beautiful and phys-ically fit women, and all of them looked fantastic.

Even the most physically fit professional athletes have different body weights at different ages and stages of life. One male pro basketball player I knew played at 190 pounds in college but weighed 220 when he played in the pros. Now, at age forty-five, he weighs 235 and is still healthy, extremely active, and very attractive.

The moral? We must expand our definition of beauty and reject cultural standards that make millions of beautiful and perfectly normal people feel overweight and unattractive. Each of us is unique, and pursuing a single, culturally created ideal of beauty is dangerous and self-defeating. Instead, let your body naturally shed its excess weight and discover your own individual beauty.

Putting It All Together

By taking a realistic look at your genetic background, the typical body shape and size of your family members, your age and hormonal status, and your BMI, you can create a fitness goal that's right for you and healthy for your body. As you do, remember that there are no "one size fits all" rules that dictate your ideal weight. Each of us is one of a kind, and trying to transform your body into your favorite fashion model's body is as unrealistic as expecting your Siamese cat to turn into a Manx.

So if you're a serial dieter, throw away your mental images of fashion models' bodies or Schwarzenegger muscles, accept and respect the body you own, and make it your goal to shape that body into a trim, healthy body—not the sad, starved body that Hollywood wants you to have. And if you've given up altogether on achieving the body you desire, and you've resigned yourself to a life of obesity, get excited! It's time to realize that long-term weight loss and health can be yours, because it's the combination of unnatural cultural goals and counterproductive dieting that made you overweight—and rejecting both of these toxic influences will free you to lose weight and attain the body you want.

Step Three: Decide That You Are Good Enough Today to Love Yourself Today

"If an individual is able to love productively, he loves himself too; if he can love only others, he cannot love at all."

Psychologist Erich Fromm[1]

I was twenty-four years old and unhappy with my body. After years of dieting, I'd gained twenty-five pounds. I felt empty and ugly, trapped in a thick and unfeminine shape that no one could love.

Sometimes I shopped for clothes, but I avoided any bold or sexy outfits. I was convinced that I was too huge to look attractive. Frequently I bought clothes a size too small, unwilling to accept my weight and myself.

One night a friend lured me out of my shell and took me to a bar in Green-wich Village. Nursing a drink, I glanced at another table and saw a handsome man talking to a woman. He was leaning close to her, seemingly mesmerized. She was shorter than me but about the same weight. (Of course, that was the first thing I noticed.) She wore a tight-fitting shirt that showed off her cleavage, and I picked up a trace of Chanel. Her diamond earrings twinkled in the light from the candle between them.

As I watched the two, totally focused on each other, I realized something: She was desirable. She was sexy. She turned him on. Her beauty showed on the outside, not because she was model thin but because she cared for herself. Her beauty stemmed from her love of herself, which was her own and grew from within.

YOU'VE BEEN TOLD all your life that weight loss is all about calories, carbohydrates, exercise, and self-denial. Eat less, exercise harder, get fit. As Tina Turner would say, "What's love got to do with it?"

The answer is very simple: *self-love is the most powerful weight-loss tool you possess.* Ironically, to achieve and sustain long-term weight loss, you must first love yourself now, exactly the way you are. When you do this, you will begin to break the patterns that made you gain excess weight in the first place and that make this weight so difficult for you to lose.

One of the most damaging aspects of food and body image preoccupation is that it creates the sense that "who I am today is unlovable and unacceptable, but the person I will be when I achieve an ideal body weight will be lovable and acceptable." You buy into this destructive belief anytime you say to yourself:

"I'll buy myself some new clothes when I lose some weight."
"I'll find a better relationship after I lose weight."
"I'll start working out at the gym after I lose weight."
"I'll take up tennis when I lose weight."

This idea—that only when you achieve a certain body size will you buy new clothes, date, travel, use sexy perfume, go to a public pool, play tennis—is based on the belief, reinforced unforgivingly by a weight-obsessed culture, that you are unworthy of these things until you have the "ideal" body. It is as if you should be so ashamed of yourself for your perceived imperfections that you deny yourself the experience of life itself. Living your life in the grip of this belief forces you into a self-destructive catch-22. In addition to starving yourself physically as you diet, you starve yourself of affection, adding unbearable emotional hunger to unbearable physical hunger. Like an abusive parent telling a child, "You're a terrible, worthless person," you may tell yourself every day that you are not worthy of love, not worthy of joy, not even worthy of a ten-dollar bottle of perfume or a trip to the pool. And where does all of this self-criticism and self-denial lead? Right to the refrigerator!

> *"My son has no life outside his work," a distressed mother told me recently. "He keeps saying, 'I'll start looking for a relationship after I lose forty pounds.' Do you know how many years he's been saying that? And he just keeps getting heavier."*

If we cannot provide for our own needs, our minds and bodies will do what is necessary to be sure we feel safe and loved. If we cannot nurture ourselves in healthy ways, we will seek more primitive means of comforting ourselves, and the most primitive and powerful comfort is food.

Have you ever dieted for weeks, refusing to buy yourself a new pair of jeans or go to a nightclub or other social gathering until you were "thin enough" and then binged on an entire carton of ice cream or a whole pizza? Or turned down a date or an outing to the movies with friends because you were "too fat" and then devoured a loaf of bread? Or followed a diet religiously for weeks and then, giving in to your desire for "forbidden" foods, thrown in the towel and quickly gained back the weight you lost—and more? Or given up entirely on weight loss, believing yourself to be too weak-willed to be fit and attractive and resigning yourself to a life of overeating and excess weight?

If so, you probably felt weak, out of control, even as though you were a bad person. But it wasn't your eating that was unnatural; it was the lack of self-love that led to the eating. What you were doing, in reality, was responding to a desperate inner cry for nurturing and love—in any form.

What I want you to do is simple: *start listening to that cry for help.*

The act of bingeing or overeating often is a cry against our aloneness, an unconscious regression back to our first human connection, that of being nursed and nurtured by our mothers. When we eat the foods that comfort us, we revisit the primordial pleasure of feeding, of being cared for, of bonding with another loving human being. We eat not because we are weak or bad but because we have no other means, at that time, of loving ourselves and healing our pain.

To end the destructive pattern of starving and bingeing, it is first necessary to answer our need for love—and that love must begin with self-love and self-acceptance. If a child cries out for help or love, you respond with open arms. Can you picture yourself saying to that child, "I'm sorry, but I don't love and accept you today, because you're too fat and I think you're disgusting—but try again when you're thinner"? It is every bit as destructive to send this unforgiving and hateful message to yourself, and the day you stop is the day you will begin on the path to becoming both mentally and physically fit and losing your excess weight forever.

Unlearning Negative Self-Talk

To learn to truly love and accept yourself, you must first become aware of the unloving and self-critical messages you send yourself each day—messages that actively hurt you and can make you turn to food to bandage your self-inflicted wounds. This is hard for most of us, because these messages are so ingrained, so habitual, that they barely register consciously.

To hear them, listen carefully to your own thoughts. Notice if you find yourself sending these messages:

"I have ugly thighs."
"I look so gross."
"I can't go out looking like this."
"I don't really need/deserve this new jacket."
"My sister is so much prettier than I am."
"The other guys at the gym must laugh at me every time I come in—I look so flabby next to them."
"I hate all this disgusting fat on my stomach."
"I can't believe I ate an entire box of Thin Mints. There's something wrong with me. I'm repulsive."

Again, picture saying any of these hurtful things to a child or to your best friend. Imagine turning to a little boy or girl who's skipping down the street and saying, "Oh, my—don't you have an ugly, fat belly?" or telling your mother or father, "I hate looking at your big butt. You're grotesque. Why do you think you should eat that hamburger?"

Would saying these things help them? Would it inspire them? Would it make their lives better? Would it motivate them to improve? Or would it cause them terrible shame and pain and lead them straight to the comfort of a food binge?

Carol Bloom and her colleagues, who treat women with eating disorders, call the chronic self-criticism of dieters "trashing." "Trashing is central to all eating problems," they say. "It completely dominates any compassion [dieters] might have for themselves. . . . Trashing can be loud and blatant—'I'm such a fat pig, slob, wild, and out of control'—or subtle, a slight internal disruption manifest when the [dieter] compares herself to others and feels diminished or uncomfortable." No matter which form the self-criticism takes, they say, it is part of a self-perpetuating cycle: "Dieting leads to bingeing, so bingeing leads to trashing, and trashing leads to more bingeing or dieting."[2]

Each time you find yourself thinking such negative thoughts about yourself, imagine a large red stop sign. Also, if possible, write down each negative thought and then, at the end of the day, review the negative messages you've been sending yourself. Again, imagine saying the same negative words out loud, to a person for whom you care deeply, or imagine how upset you would feel if you heard your good friends saying these things about themselves. Now imagine being as kind to yourself as you are to others. One statement I find myself making again and again in the process of providing therapy for a myriad of psychiatric problems is "Actively work on being as kind to yourself as you would to another who has walked in your shoes."

At first this may seem strange, because you're probably used to being very harsh with yourself. Eventually, however, you will find it easier and easier to rephrase your inner dialogues in a kind way. If this is very hard for you, you may find it helpful to talk with an understanding therapist. (I also recommend a wonderful book, *Feeling Good: The New Mood Therapy*, by Dr. David Burns.)

As you become increasingly aware of negative self-talk, practice rephrasing your inner dialogue in a way that is less abusive. (For instance, if you're a woman, try saying to yourself, "My thighs are soft and rounded" rather than "I have fat thighs." If you're a man, try saying, "I have my dad's build" rather than "I'm too large.") Similarly, when you look at yourself in the mirror, look at yourself with affection and compassion, just as you would look at a loved one. When you do, you will be amazed at the psychic energy you free up to pursue your goals and the lessening of the burden you carry.

Just how powerful can the act of relinquishing self-criticism be? In *The Obsession: Reflections on the Tyranny of Slenderness*, Kim Chernin writes of the experience of looking at herself in the mirror without hating what she saw: "For the first time I was able to perceive the transparent film of expectation I placed over my image in the looking glass. I had never seen myself before. Until now, all I had been able to behold was my body's failure to conform to an ideal. Now, I realized that what I had called fat in myself, and considered gross, was this body of a woman. And it was beautiful."

You, too, are beautiful or handsome in your own, individual way. Becoming able to realize this, and allowing yourself to love and nurture the beauty that is within you, will take active energy on your part. By doing so, you will empower yourself, and that power will allow you to achieve your goals. Remind yourself, each time you find yourself being self-critical, that your ideas about your body's "wrongness" are a result of a lifelong process of cultural brainwashing that has convinced you that an unnaturally thin body is a necessary component of beauty—just as people in other times were brainwashed to believe that only pink skin was beautiful or that binding women's feet to make them unnaturally small made the women more attractive.

But doesn't accepting yourself as you are mean that you will no longer be motivated to change, if you truly do need to lose weight and become more fit? No! It is legitimate to want to change and improve, and we are in fact changing all the time, whether we want to or not. If you are overweight, losing weight and accepting the process of change is a positive action that will enhance your life. But positive transformation, including the act of losing excess weight, begins with self-acceptance. In accepting both ourselves and our needs, we also learn to satiate those needs. We learn that we are not bottomless pits of want and that we can feel loved and full and satisfied without being self-destructive.

This is what I want you to recognize: that *you are not your weight*. Neither are you a "bad" person or a person who is weak or out of control. You are a dignified, complex, emotional being, wrestling with a problem—whether it's excess weight, repetitive dieting, overeating, binge eating, or bulimia—that can be solved. Think of this problem as being like the worn carpets and faded paint in a well-loved house. It may be a significant problem, but it doesn't affect the fact that the house is a wonderful building that shelters and protects you. And just as the house can be repaired and repainted in a loving way, so can you begin to change yourself with love and self-acceptance.

Years ago, at a time when I still cringed every time I looked in a mirror, I sat watching rock videos on TV one day with my nephew. I wasn't paying much attention, just letting the music wash over me. Then a song came on, and the repetitive lyrics and sensual dancing filtered through my daydreams.

The lyrics, sung over and over again, said: "Shake what your mamma gave you, shake what your mamma gave you!" The lyrics immediately resonated within me, because they contrasted so dramatically with what I'd been pro-grammed to believe: that I could take what I wanted, do what I wanted to do, say what I wanted to say, and be what I wanted to be only if I fit into an impos-sible mold. To me the lyrics were offering the opposite message: "Take what you are and what you have and use it to be all you can be. Enjoy the beat of life with as much energy and passion as you can find within you."

Some of my friends and students laugh when I tell them, but to this day I find inspiration in "Shake what your mamma gave you!" When I'm supervising intel-ligent young medical students, and I see them hesitating to give an answer to a question, or afraid to jump in with an opinion, I tell them about that rap song. They look at me strangely, but they get the message—and the next time around, they are less afraid to believe in themselves.

Author Marianne Williamson once said, "Our deepest fear is not that we are inadequate. Our deepest fear is that we are powerful beyond measure. It is our light, not our darkness, that most frightens us. We ask ourselves, 'Who am I to be brilliant, gorgeous, talented, fabulous?' Actually, who are you NOT to be? You are a child of God. Your playing small does not serve the world. . . . As we let our light shine, we give others permission to do the same."

Seeing Through Your Excuses

One effect of dieting and our unwillingness to love ourselves in the present is that it makes us lie to ourselves and to others. When we deny ourselves opportunities to connect to others or participate in life, because we believe we are not acceptable enough to deserve or participate in the experiences, we often make excuses. For instance, we may say:

"I'm just too tired to go to the beach with you." (Translation: "I look fat and ugly in a swimsuit, but I'll go with you when I'm a size 12.")

"I'd join your bowling league, but the boss has me working too much over-time." (Translation: "None of you are overweight, and I don't want to be the 'fat guy' on the team.")

"I'd love to go on that cruise, but I can't afford it." (Translation: "Cruises are for attractive people, and I'm not attractive now.")

"I'll have to pass on the mall today—there's so much housework I should do." (Translation: "I'm not buying myself new clothes until I lose thirty pounds.")

These excuses keep us stuck in our destructive patterns, because to change a behavior, it is necessary to understand it. If you find yourself inventing reasons for not doing what you want or buying yourself what you desire, ask yourself: "Why am I saying no to an experience I'd love to enjoy or to a gift I'd love to give myself?"

If those excuses are covering up the belief that you don't deserve the experience because of your weight, then it's critical that you become aware of what you're doing and how it's hurting you and resolve to base your decisions on self-love rather than self-criticism. And if you avoid these activities out of shame about your weight, consider studying the impact this deprivation is having in your life.

I ask you to live your life today as you would if you were already at your perceived ideal weight. In doing so, you are actively helping yourself lose weight.

Love Is an Action

Saying that you love yourself is a first step toward healing and toward permanent weight loss. But to truly overcome the self-criticism caused by years of dieting, you need to *act on your love*. As Erich Fromm says, "The capacity to love demands a state of intensity, awakeness, enhanced vitality, which can only be the result of productive and active orientation."[3] That means being actively concerned about your own interests, your own needs, and your own well-being.

Caroline grew up in a family where she experienced full and unconditional love from her mother. Her father, however, was a different story. He was very unpre-dictable, and Caroline's mother called him a "fair-weather father." She would tell Caroline, "Your father may say terrible things, but he really loves you." Car-oline's mother used the same rationale in her own relationship with him, even though at times he was cruel and disrespectful.

What did this teach Caroline? If she could convince herself that someone really did love her, then she could accept being treated poorly. This led, predictably, to a series of unhealthy and hurtful relationships. Eventually, after therapy, Caroline learned to hold those who love her accountable not only for their feelings toward her but also for their actions toward her. This led her to much more fulfilling relationships and a stable life where her needs are met.

Caroline learned that she had a choice: she could accept cruelty from others, or she could expect other people to treat her well. The same principle applies to how we treat ourselves. We can actually make a *choice* to treat ourselves with love and dignity. We don't need to wait for some magical moment to occur—for instance, when we lose a dress size. We can instead choose to love ourselves, very much, the way we currently are. By doing so, we open the door to a happier life, in which we no longer need to turn to food to comfort ourselves and assuage our pain.

This means more, however, than simply saying "I love myself." It means *acting* on that belief, by treating ourselves as lovingly as we treat others. As M. Scott Peck says, in *The Road Less Traveled*, "Genuine love is volitional rather than emotional. The person who truly loves does so because of a decision to love. This person has made a commitment to be loving whether or not the loving feeling is present. . . . True love is not a feeling by which we are overwhelmed. It is a committed, thoughtful decision."

Peck stresses that this active love to which we should aspire includes self-love: "We are incapable of loving another unless we love ourselves. . . . We cannot be a source of strength unless we nurture our own strength."

What does this mean in terms of day-to-day behavior? It means that you must begin to treat yourself with dignity as a delicate and special being. You must forgive yourself for your imperfections and be as kind to yourself as you are to your friends and family. And it means that you must accept the responsibility of caring for your own needs, just as you take responsibility for the needs of others. In this sense responsibility implies "being responsive"—listening to your needs and being able and ready to respond to them.

This may mean buying yourself new clothes. It may mean saving up for the cruise you've been dreaming of taking, buying some makeup, getting a massage, or putting on your swimsuit and going to the beach.

At first these simple actions may seem foreign or even selfish. That's because men and women who fall into the trap of compulsive dieting often are "people pleasers," whose lives revolve around satisfying others while neglecting themselves. We are so accustomed to focusing our energies on meeting the needs of boyfriends, girlfriends, spouses, children, or parents that many of us actually need to train ourselves to say, "What do I want? What do I need?"

The effort, however, is well worth it. When you learn to love yourself, and to care for yourself and your own needs, you will begin to live in the moment, a rich moment in which you can dream for the future while savoring exactly who and where you are today. And that is the first huge step out of the prison of dieting and self-hatred and into the happy life you deserve.

A Word About Perfectionism

Many of us who develop food and weight preoccupations are high achievers—and yet, because of our drive for perfection, we never feel "good enough."

In a limited sense, the urge to achieve perfection is a healthy drive. But when the goal ceases to be "I want to be better at what I do" and instead becomes "I must be perfect at everything I do," perfectionism breeds low self-esteem. That's because absolute perfection is an impossible goal, and anyone who strives for that goal will fail.

Some of us are more vulnerable to the tyranny of perfectionism than others. High-risk individuals include:

- men and women in professions that place excessive emphasis on outward appearance—for instance, acting or modeling
- athletes of either sex, particularly those involved in bodybuilding
- "good girls" and high-achieving boys who spend their lives pleasing and placating others
- young gay men

Anyone, however, can suffer from perfectionism so extreme that it becomes crippling. If you are a perfectionist, you may need to work at becoming aware of the impossible standards you set for yourself and the punishment you inflict on yourself for your perceived failures. It will take energy and concentration to pay attention to the negative scripts you play in your head if you binge or exceed your self-imposed calorie limits or exercise less than you think is necessary. And consider the limiting role that perfectionism plays in the rest of your life as well. Do you refuse to go out in public dressed in attractive clothes, because your body is larger than you want it to be? Do you turn down dates with people you find attractive, because you think they'll reject you for not being "good enough"?

If so, what might happen if you focused instead on allowing yourself to be human rather than perfect? When you release yourself from the need for perfection, you are likely to discover a tremendous freedom and sense of well-being. You may find that your horizons expand, and your focus on food becomes less important, when you learn to accept the idea that being human means being unique, interesting, and sometimes flawed—not being inhumanly perfect.

Take the Time to "Look at" and "Know" Yourself: An Exercise in Self-Respect and Self-Discovery

The Latin root of the word *respect* is *respicere*, literally "to look at." The word *conscious* derives from the Latin *scire*, meaning "to know." As you follow this fitness plan, make it your goal to respect and become conscious of yourself, in the true definition of these words. Realizing your potential means seeing what is special, unique, and beautiful about yourself and learning to know, love, admire, and respect yourself just as you are—not next month or next year but today.

When you accomplish this goal, you will discover that losing excess weight becomes far easier. To lose weight effectively and permanently, you must learn to be sensitive to yourself. When you do, you will be able to concentrate on yourself and your needs and address these needs in positive and loving ways rather than masking them with food. And you will learn to live your life in the present, fully and joyously, rather than postponing your existence until a day when you are "good enough."

So make a vow, today, to become conscious of your self-denial and to love yourself actively and treat yourself kindly. Use the exercises at the end of this chapter to increase your awareness of the pain that self-criticism causes you and to change this destructive pattern into a life-affirming pattern that will put you on the path to healthy weight loss and a happier life.

Make a commitment to do the first two activities every day. Remember: emotional change takes work and commitment!

Existence Without Activity

To lose weight, you must learn to love yourself—and a critical step in learning to love yourself is learning to simply *be with* yourself.

At first, the following exercise may seem strange or uncomfortable, simply because our "do-oriented" culture trains us to be in motion constantly and to solve every problem by *doing* rather than *being*. But as you become aware of your eating, you may realize that you often eat when you are bored, lonely, or anxious. The purpose of this exercise is to enable you to tolerate these states and to tolerate being alone, without turning to food to "fill" yourself. As a result, this simple exercise will do far more to help you lose weight than all of the energy and labor you've put into dieting.

Set aside fifteen minutes each day to do nothing other than concentrate on yourself. Ask your friends and family to leave you alone during this time and find a quiet place where you feel relaxed. At the end of the concentration exercise, make notes describing what you recall about the experience. How did it feel? Were you anxious? Comfortable? What was the content of your thoughts? In what ways were your thoughts kind to you? In what ways were they unkind?

The importance of this concentration exercise cannot be overstated. This is a time when your mind and body are connected and a time to examine the thoughts flowing through your mind. It is a time to practice doing *nothing* and to become comfortable simply "being." This activity teaches you to listen to your body and respect its messages. In addition, it teaches you how to enjoy the experience of being alone with yourself, just as you would enjoy being with another person you love. The ability to tolerate aloneness is an essential step in the process of recognizing your inner state—and acknowledging your inner needs and feelings, in turn, is a crucial step toward differentiating between true hunger and non-hunger-based eating.

Self-Denial Inventory

Each day, make a list of the activities that filled your day. How could you have made your day more pleasurable? In what ways did you deny yourself enjoyable experiences or desired things?

Make a list of five things you haven't done because of your concerns about your weight or your body.

_____

_____

_____

_____

_____

Make a list of the reasons you gave yourself or others for not participating in activities or for denying yourself things that you wanted. For example: "I don't have enough money," "I need to get some work done," "My house is a mess."

_____

_____

_____

_____

_____

_____

When you denied yourself things that you desired or did not allow yourself to participate in activities you would have enjoyed, what did you do instead?

_____

_____

_____

_____

_____

_____

Close your eyes and picture yourself participating in activities you enjoy or giving yourself the gifts you have denied yourself. Now imagine what would have happened if you had allowed yourself to experience these pleasurable activities or to enjoy the items you denied yourself.

As an additional part of this step, think of something you've promised to buy for yourself as soon as you lose weight. If you can afford it, *buy it the next time you go out.* Preferably, make it something sexy, fun, or outrageous—not something practical.

Journal Writing

Erich Fromm notes that "love is an art, just as living is an art; if we want to learn how to love we must proceed in the same way we have to proceed if we want to learn any other art, say music, painting, carpentry, or the art of medicine or engineering."[4]

The same philosophy applies to loving yourself: once you realize the need to love yourself, it is necessary to *practice the art* of loving yourself. As part of this practice, begin a journal. Each day, write down the loving acts you performed for yourself. Do not be critical of yourself if you skip a day of writing or if you have no self-loving acts to record. The purpose of your journal is to increase your awareness of your acts of self-criticism or self-love and gently guide you toward respecting and loving yourself.

Part III

Steps Four
Through Seven

*Take Action: Solve Your Weight
Problems Permanently*

IN STEPS FOUR through Seven, I'll ask you to transform the insight you've gained into action. You will learn how to face food every day in a way that is true to yourself and your needs, while promoting long-term health and weight management.

These steps literally teach you to relearn your relationship with food, helping you rediscover your natural ability to achieve a healthy weight and attractive body without dieting—an ability stolen from you by a culture that falsely believes that dieting is the key to weight loss.

You'll also reevaluate the role of exercise in your life and learn how expanding your definition of exercise (and throwing away the misguided idea that exercise has to hurt or bore you) can enhance your ability to become fit and lose excess pounds. In addition, you'll learn how to get *real* help from your doctor—not just another lecture and a diet plan but evaluations that can remove any medical barriers to weight loss.

As you relearn your relationship with food and your body, you'll discover a new diet-free, guilt-free, and self-preserving path to lifelong fitness. When you follow these steps, your excess pounds will begin to disappear for good and you will discover that it *is* possible to achieve your weight-loss goals, while enjoying a relaxed relationship with food.

Step Four: Learn to Experience, Trust, and Enjoy Hunger and Satiation

"Forget will power, discipline, and self control. . . . Eat when you are hungry and stop eating when the hunger is satisfied. We were all born with the ability to do this until diets, clocks and people told us what to eat, when to eat and how much to eat."

Registered dietitian Noreen Williams[1]

IN THIS STEP I'm asking you to do something that you probably believe is impossible: I'm asking you to trust yourself.

As a former repetitive dieter, I know just how terrifying this step is. As a recovered dieter and a medical doctor, however, I also know that *it's the single most crucial step toward a healthy, fit, attractive body and lasting weight loss.* This one step—trusting your hunger—is the key to freeing yourself from food anxiety, guilt, self-criticism, and enslavement to an endless string of diets that end in weight gain and despair. *It is the way out.*

Before you begin this step, however, it's important to understand what's at stake. Think about the reasons you picked up this book in the first place. Think about the days, weeks, and years you've sacrificed to diets that didn't work. Think about the parties and holiday meals and brunches and dinner dates you've dreaded; the "forbidden" foods that you crave; the binges you can't control; the sinking feeling when you step on the scale each morning; and the toll that food preoccupation takes on your energy, your self-esteem, and your dreams for the future.

Are you happy repeating, over and over again, the cycle of perpetual dieting and perpetual weight gain? Will you be happy living this way for another ten, twenty, or thirty years? Will you feel fulfilled and happy if your life centers forever on calories, carbohydrates, diet pills, diet drinks, and numbers on a bathroom scale—and you keep gaining more and more weight?

If not, it's time to say "No more." When an approach to a problem fails over and over and over again, and medical science tells you that it will continue to fail each time you try it, it's time to look for a new solution. And when it comes to dieting, the only real solution is to stop the madness—the madness of yo-yo dieting that causes you to gain twice as much weight as you lose—and try a new and better approach to weight loss. To stop dieting, however, you must learn to start eating when your body tells you to eat and learn to recognize when you are satiated.

Kelly came to me for help in losing weight. A smart and attractive thirty-six-year-old advertising executive, she'd gained ten pounds after her first pregnancy. She lost the weight on a nine-hundred-calorie-a-day liquid diet, but when she quit the diet she put on twenty pounds. After three more babies and dozens of failed diets, Kelly—now forty pounds heavier than the day she started dieting—desperately needed a solution. "I hate my body," she said, "and everything I try makes it worse."

Kelly and I talked about her eating patterns. She told me that she ate a small breakfast early each morning, even though she wasn't particularly hungry. "By eleven I am hungry," she said, "but I don't eat then, because I tell myself it's only an hour until lunchtime."

At twelve-thirty each day, Kelly headed for a buffet restaurant, with every intention of eating a salad and a bowl of soup. "Some days I can do it," she told me. "But other days I look at all of this food surrounding me—puddings, muffins, potato salad, chicken-fried steak and gravy—and I just can't stop myself. It's like I'll never be able to eat enough to feel full."

As I listened, thoughts of my own dieting days surfaced in my mind. I remembered telling my own therapist, years earlier, about my binges. "I can't stop," I'd said. "I don't know why I can't control myself."

I'd expected her to ask deep questions: Why did I feel that I couldn't control myself? What triggered my binges? Instead she'd startled me by responding with a simple question:

"What do you eat for breakfast?"

When I answered—a hard-boiled egg, an apple, a slice of dry toast—she nodded, unsurprised. She didn't see my bingeing as an act of uncontrolled gluttony. She recognized it as my body's natural response to hunger denied.

Nothing is simpler than eating when you're hungry and stopping when you're satiated. Babies know this. They cry, fuss, and search for their mother's breast when they crave food. Once they eat enough, they turn their heads, sated and content. They don't starve, they don't binge, and they don't have weight problems.

As I noted in Chapter 2, diets replace hunger-driven eating with diet-driven eating. When you diet, it doesn't matter what you want to eat or when you want to eat it. If you're hungry for pancakes at ten o'clock, you tell yourself "no" and eat cottage cheese at noon instead. Or you eat a banana instead of the pancakes. Or you make pancakes with sugar-free syrup and then go without lunch, even though you're starving again by two o'clock.

When you continually ignore your hunger in this manner, suppressing your inner drives and forcing your body to follow an artificial timetable, you decouple your appetite from your eating. The results:

- You no longer eat when you're hungry, because you no longer recognize the sensation of hunger.

- You no longer *stop* eating when your body should feel full, because you cannot recognize the signals that say "enough."

As a result, you become trapped in a cycle of dieting and weight gain. To break this pattern of unsuccessful dieting, you need to learn again how to recognize and respond to your inner feelings of hunger and satiation, just as you did when you were a child. And to do this, you first need to learn to listen to your body and your feelings.

I asked Kelly to begin her days with the concentration exercise I described in Step Three. Each morning she spent fifteen minutes in a peaceful setting, paying attention to her thoughts, her feelings, and how her body felt.

At first Kelly said, "It's so hard. I keep thinking about my financial problems. I tell myself, 'Stop—you're not supposed to be worrying about bills and credit cards right now'—but I can't seem to turn it off and just relax."

I asked Kelly to think about what she'd just said. Was there a reason her mind kept returning to her money problems? And didn't it make more sense to listen to her concerns and fears, rather than simply saying "no" to them?

As we talked, Kelly realized that she needed to respect her own thoughts and feelings. In particular, she recognized that she needed to communicate more with her husband and together develop a plan for addressing their financial problems to resolve the issues that troubled her during her morning concentration sessions.

Similarly, Kelly eventually began to realize that when her body signaled, "I'm hungry," she should listen to it, no matter what a diet book or a clock said. She realized that saying "no" to her hunger didn't make it go away. Instead it made her so desperate for food that by the time she reached the buffet line no amount of willpower could counter her body's urge to overeat.

Kelly began taking snacks to work—not just carrot sticks or rice cakes but filling and satisfying snacks that she enjoyed—and eating them at midmorning when she felt hungry. The result: when she went to lunch, she was no longer ravenous, and her "buffet binges" gradually became a thing of the past.

Kelly felt out of control at the buffet for a simple reason: she ignored her inner messages. When we ignore normal hunger, it becomes ravenous hunger, leading to overeating and weight gain. To understand why, it's important to understand how hunger works and why it's so dangerous to ignore your hunger signals.

Your body possesses remarkable biological computers that constantly calculate your glucose and hormone levels, the levels of amino acids and fats in your systems, and even your body temperature. The tiny hypothalamus in the brain uses these data to generate sensations that tell you, "It's time to eat." When you eat, similar mechanisms eventually tell you, "That's enough—you're full and you don't desire any more food right now." Like the players in an orchestra, your body's chemicals—cortisol, cholecystokinin, insulin, estrogen, neuropeptide Y, serotonin, norepinephrine, dopamine, and many more—work together, creating the natural inner music of hunger and satiation.

Diets, however, teach you to be tone-deaf to the signals your body sends. Diets teach you that it's wrong to eat a morning snack, to be hungry right before bedtime, or to crave pasta when you're supposed to eat steamed vegetables. Diets teach you that there are right and wrong times to eat and right and wrong foods to eat—and they teach you that you must stop eating when you finish an "allowed" portion, even if you're still hungry. When you buy into these myths, you learn to suppress your awareness of your hunger and satiation signals, until eventually you cannot hear them. Your unacknowledged hunger grows and grows, until when you do allow yourself to eat you find it hard—sometimes impossible—to stop.

To picture this process, imagine your hunger as a smoke alarm ringing in your home. If you listen and respond, you can put the fire out when it's still small and easy to smother. But if you ignore the alarm and allow the fire to grow, it will become an all-consuming, unstoppable blaze. In the same way, ignored hunger grows and grows, becoming raging, unquenchable hunger. As a result you become convinced that your appetite is insatiable, and you become trapped in the process of repetitive dieting.

I know the pattern all too well. Like Kelly, I constantly denied my hunger when I dieted. When low-cal diets were the rage, I lived on a thousand calories a day. When fasting diets came into vogue, I lived on broth and carrot juice. If a diet book said, "Don't eat any food after dinner," I gave up evening snacks. And all of my efforts, like Kelly's, led inexorably to more binges and more gained pounds.

Many people find this dieting-and-overeating cycle so psychically and physically damaging that they give up altogether, believing that a life of being overweight is less agonizing than a life of alternating starvation and out-of-control eating. Many others continue to follow the same no-win scenario of dieting and to blame themselves as each diet fails them. Whatever group we fall into, we continue to believe that our hunger is "bad" and "wrong" and that we are weak for giving in to it.

To overcome my diet-and-binge pattern, I had to learn to take my hunger seriously. I had to listen to my body and respect its wisdom. And that is what you, too, must do, to break the cycle of dieting, bingeing, or overeating and achieve true fitness and health.

Are You an "Emotional Grazer"?

In Step Four, I'm asking you to fully trust your feelings of hunger and satiation. To do this, you'll need to give up the bad habits that dieting teaches you. In addition, however, you may need to spot and break ingrained patterns that cause you to use food as a substitute for other needs.

As you learn to eat naturally, following the points I outline in this chapter, it's also important to become conscious of the reasons that you eat. For instance:

- Does food substitute for a mother, father, lover, or best friend in your life?
- Are you stuck in a rut, emotionally or professionally, and using food to avoid facing your loneliness or boredom?
- Does eating ease your anxiety or help you avoid facing fears about the future?
- Does eating reduce your restlessness when you are sedentary?

Any of these hidden motivations can lead to obesity due to "emotional grazing," a pattern of eating almost unconsciously and without any relation to hunger. Sometimes we're vulnerable to grazing at certain times of day, with certain individuals, or in certain situations. (For instance, after a stressful day, many of us eat a full dinner and then sit in front of the television munching on ice cream, caramel corn, potato chips, or any other snack that comes to hand, almost without being aware of the state of our bodies—a way of numbing ourselves emotionally through eating.)

As you eat naturally, try to recognize the triggers that make you eat when you're not hungry and ask yourself: What purpose is the food serving in my life? Are there other ways to satisfy this need? For help in identifying your unmet needs, and in discovering positive ways to satisfy them, read Step Three (Decide That You Are Good Enough Today to Love Yourself Today), Step Five (Straight Talk About Exercise), and Step Nine (Redefine Your Life: What's More Important to You Than Dieting?).

"But I'm Afraid"

So was I. I dieted for years because I believed that if I ate whatever I wanted, I'd never stop.

After decades of dieting, the idea of eating without a diet plan left me paralyzed with fear. I pictured a diet-free life as a perpetual binge, because I couldn't imagine gaining control over my appetite. (Another woman told me that when she contemplated living without dieting, "I kept picturing those eight-hundred-pound people in *Ripley's Believe It or Not*. I knew if I ate whatever I wanted, I'd wind up like that.") If you've dieted for years, you probably have the same fears.

In reality, however, this is what will happen when you begin trusting and enjoying your own hunger:

• **At first you will crave "forbidden" foods, and you may eat large quantities of them.** *This stage is temporary.* You've ignored your internal messages of hunger and satiety for so long that it will take you time to learn to eat naturally. Be prepared for the fact that you may gain some weight at first and be patient. *This is not failure*—it is a necessary and expected step toward overcoming your diet mentality and achieving long-term weight loss. If you eat a pint of peaches-and-cream ice cream every day for a week, or devour three Big Macs at one sitting, that's an understandable reaction to chronic deprivation. Realize that this brief phase is a stepping-stone from dieting to diet-free weight loss and that it will pass.

• **As you continue to allow yourself to eat, food will lose its control over you.** Right now you crave chocolate cake or stuffing or lemon meringue pie because you denied yourself these foods for years or tormented yourself with guilt when you ate them. When these foods are no longer off-limits, and you can eat them anytime you want them, as long as you're hungry—for breakfast, lunch, and dinner, if you like!—they will lose the magical power that dieting conferred on them. (Sometimes, in fact, you'll find that you don't like them at all.)

For years I craved bread and refused to allow it in my house. When I first started eating the foods I loved, I devoured massive amounts of French bread, muffins, and buttered rolls. At first these foods tasted like ambrosia to me. Within a few weeks, however, I reached the point where bread was simply bread, and a slice or two satisfied me completely. Similarly, a friend of mine craved Twinkies and Hostess cupcakes. After she began eating them again, she told me, "Now I remember why I got sick of them when I was a kid."

Like us, as you learn to sense your hunger, respond to that hunger, and freely choose the foods you desire, you'll discover that "forbidden fruit" is infinitely less attractive when it's no longer forbidden. Without the mystique of being taboo, a Twinkie is just a Twinkie.

• **When you eat naturally, you will be satisfied and in control.** Dieting short-circuits the biological signals that tell you that you're full. Even worse, it short-circuits your psychological sense of satiation, because it forbids you to eat enough to satisfy your hunger and tells you that you can't eat the foods you desire, creating an insatiable desire for them. When you overcome these unnatural physical and mental barriers to satiation, you will no longer lose control when you eat.

• **As you satisfy your cravings, you'll eventually want to eat healthy foods.** "Won't I get sick," my patients ask me, "if I eat nothing but junk?" Unless you have a health problem that requires you to restrict certain foods, the answer is no. At first you'll almost undoubtedly crave salty or fried or sugary foods. But when you get your fill of these foods, your body will naturally begin to crave good foods as well. (Just as cake loses its luster when you can eat it every day, salad starts to look better when you don't *have* to eat it.) In fact, after a few months, most ex-dieters eat far more healthily than they did when they lived on unbalanced low-carb, low-protein, or no-fruit diets, followed inevitably by binges.

Remember, too, that *dieting itself is bad for your health.* Dieting can actually exacerbate health problems caused by being overweight, since studies show that diets fail 95 to 97 percent of the time and often lead to weight *gain.* Weight cycling harms your body too; as I noted in Chapter 2, yo-yo dieting is linked to osteoporosis, depression, heart problems, possibly even cancer. Dieting is a disease that can hurt both your mind and your body, and the best step you can take to protect your health is to recognize the truth about the outcome of diets and stop dieting.

Learning to identify and satiate your hunger is a necessary step in your effort to attain the body you desire and to maintain long-term weight control. When you learn to eat naturally, you will not end up fat. You will not lose control of your eating forever. Instead, over the long run, you will lose the weight you gained from yo-yo dieting and almost assuredly improve your long-term health—and you will free yourself from the tyranny of diets that don't work.

Before You Begin: Understanding Guilt and Dissociation

Guilt (noun) A painful feeling of self-reproach resulting from a belief that one has done something wrong or immoral. *(dictionary definition)*

Have you noticed that the word *guilt* keeps cropping up throughout this book? That's because guilt is one of the biggest challenges you'll need to face and overcome as you recover from food and body preoccupation.

Our feelings about food and our bodies result from a barrage of images inflicted on us by a society that mandates unrealistic beauty ideals. When we internalize these impossible definitions of beauty, we diet in a desperate response to achieve an unachievable goal. Inevitably, however, we break our diets and eat the "bad" foods we've denied ourselves. When we do, we feel tremendous guilt—and, ironically, that guilt can lead to bingeing.

Another Reason Diets Make You Gain Weight

You went on the cabbage diet and wound up at Burger King at midnight, wolfing down a Whopper. Or you spent three weeks on a low-carb diet and then broke your diet with three helpings of spaghetti.

Lack of willpower? No. More likely your "cheats" occurred because different bodies need different foods at different times. For instance:

- Before they reach puberty, girls crave high-carbohydrate foods. Experts believe this is linked to a surge in a chemical called neuropeptide Y.

- Young boys, conversely, prefer high-protein foods, probably in response to changing levels of growth hormone factor.

- After puberty the body produces higher levels of galanin and opioids (natural neurotransmitters/neuromodulators that affect behavior, mood, pain sensation, and endocrine function). These natural substances make both males and females crave more fat in their diets. Women, whose bodies are preparing for reproduction, develop these fat cravings earlier.

- People who experience seasonal affective disorder (SAD) become depressed during the winter months, when sunlight is scarce. They also crave carbohydrates, and carbs make them feel better—possibly because a high-carbohydrate diet temporarily alters levels of the brain chemical serotonin. This may also explain the carbohydrate cravings of women with premenstrual syndrome (PMS).

- Chocolate can alter levels of the brain chemicals serotonin and dopamine, possibly easing the physical and emotional symptoms of PMS.

- People deficient in iron often crave iron-rich hamburgers and steaks, while people deficient in calcium frequently crave cheesy foods or ice cream.

The bottom line: *your body is smarter than your diet.* If you're female, and your body craves chocolate the day before your period starts, you're not going to buy it off with the steak that's "legal" on your low-carb diet. Instead you're going to eat the steak, and then probably the chocolate too, and possibly kick off a thousand-calorie binge as well. Similarly, if you're a male or female weight lifter trying to survive on a cabbage soup diet, you're going to wind up breaking your diet with a cheeseburger, because your body needs protein to build muscle. The moral: your body knows what it's doing. Listen to it, and not to the diet gurus.

How? Imagine your guilt as a wall, like the Great Wall of China: a massive, immovable barrier between you and the restricted food that you crave. You are on one side of this wall, and the restricted food is on the other side. How do you reach the other side and obtain the food you crave, when your mind and body can no longer tolerate your deprivation? By *breaking through the barrier.* How do you do this? By experiencing a phenomenon known in psychiatry as *dissociation.*

When dieters dissociate, we break through our wall of guilt by disconnecting from our thoughts and feelings and allowing our hunger to reign unchecked. The part of us that says "I deserve that" or "I want that" or "I just must eat that now" is forced to break away in our minds from the stream of thoughts created by the "dieting mind" that says "I can't, I can't, I can't." Among the feelings we may experience when the dissociation process occurs are:

- a sense of a "rush," almost like the experience of a drug high
- a temporary relief of anxiety
- a sense of losing touch with our surroundings
- a sense of emotional numbing

When we experience dissociation, we feel overwhelming relief as we give in to our drive for the unacceptable food we crave—the "rush" of breaking free. But we pay a terrible price for this splintering of our being, as our minds and bodies become further and further decoupled from each other when we are eating, and we grow further detached from our natural sensations of hunger and satiation. Moreover, as we "awaken" at the end of each period of dissociation, we feel increasing self-disgust, increasing despair and increasing guilt. In short, we set ourselves up for the next diet/binge cycle.

In addition, the powerful reinforcement of eating becomes coupled in our minds with the experience of the "rush" we feel when we eat uncontrollably. Our minds associate eating with that rush of the binge, much as Pavlov's dog learned to associate a ringing bell with food, and this association feeds our loss of control.

How can you end this vicious cycle? By recognizing the powerfully destructive force of guilt and consciously working to overcome it. Believe it or not, the guilt that you think is protecting you from eating forbidden foods actually makes it increasingly hard for you to gain control of your eating habits.

The exercise that follows will help you learn to eat without guilt and to respect your hunger and your satiation. When you learn this skill, you will no longer need to break through the barrier of guilt to eat, and your mind and body will no longer be driven to dissociate during times of feeding. As a result the power that food possesses over you will slowly dissipate, and food will become just what it is—a satisfying pleasure rather than a dangerous and taboo addiction. Consequently you will stop the cycle of dieting and weight gain and replace it with healthy weight loss and a relaxed relationship with food.

Starting Over: Three Stages to Relearn Your Relationship with Food

When you are ready to release yourself from repetitive dieting or chronic overeating, this three-stage exercise will guide you through the process of identifying, respecting, and satisfying your hunger. It's important to do the stages of the exercise in order, because each step will prepare you for the next.

Stage One: Listen to Yourself

This concentration exercise is invaluable if you tend to graze because of boredom, inactivity, or anxiety, because it teaches you how to simply *be*, without feeling the need to *do*. An essential tool in the process of achieving permanent weight loss is the skill of tolerating inactivity. To lose weight and maintain long-term weight loss, you must learn how to exist without being "busy" every moment, because the need for constant activity often translates into eating when you're not truly hungry.

Continue to do the concentration exercise I described in the last chapter. As you sit quietly for fifteen minutes, allow your thoughts to roam freely, focusing in particular on how your body feels. Are you warm or cool? Does your stomach feel full or empty? Do you feel peaceful? Energetic or tired? Tense or relaxed?

As you sit quietly, concentrate on acknowledging and respecting your feelings and the messages of your body. This will help you identify your feelings of hunger and satiation as you learn to eat freely again.

When I first stopped dieting, I found it hard to identify the physical and emotional sensations of hunger and satiety. Now I do it instinctively. The other day, for instance, I arrived home famished after a long day and heated up a small frozen enchilada dinner. I ate the food quickly, and when it was gone I noticed a sense of anxiety and a feeling of emptiness within my stomach. Stopping to analyze this sensation, I realized that the enchilada "dinner" I'd eaten resembled the size of the portions I had eaten as a dieter. Back then I would wonder, "What's wrong with me? Why do I keep breaking my diet?" As I looked at the tiny, empty frozen food container, I laughed to myself. No wonder I never felt satiated after a diet-sized meal! How could the maker of that dinner really expect an average-sized adult to feel satisfied after eating such a minuscule amount of food?

As another step in your process of self-exploration, pay attention to your feelings before, during, and after a meal of the size you typically eat when you're dieting. Do you anticipate being satisfied by your meal? As you eat it, do you enjoy it, or are you anxious about feeling hungry after you finish? When you're done, do you feel satisfied, or do you feel empty and anxious? Analyze how you feel, and how you respond to your feelings.

Also, pay attention to the "triggers" that make you want to eat. Do you reach for a candy bar after a bad experience on a date or a stressful day at work? Does the idea of a long evening at home alone send you to the refrigerator? Or do you sometimes eat when you're faced with an unpleasant task that you're trying to put off? As you begin to recognize these triggers, you will learn to differentiate physical hunger from emotional needs that can be satisfied in different ways.

You may find that you need to wait for some time to feel hunger. Be patient—your body does need food to live, so you *will* experience hunger if you wait!

What Does Hunger Feel Like?

Different people experience the sensation of hunger in different ways. Some experience a sense of hollowness or emptiness in the abdomen, accompanied by feelings of urgency and anxiety. Others identify hunger as primarily a "mouth" sensation. Here's how some of my patients describe their feelings of hunger:

- "I feel crabby, easily annoyed, irritable. I'm willing to eat almost anything that's available at the time. I feel a little desperate."
- "I feel tired."
- "My stomach starts making noises, and I feel very irritable."
- "I feel a little 'spacy' and if I get really hungry, I feel a bit weak and shaky and have trouble concentrating."
- "I feel excited, because it's been so long since I've noticed feeling hungry, and I'm excited because I now know that I can feed my hunger with something I really want without feeling guilty."
- "My stomach starts feeling like it's knotting up, and I start to feel light-headed."

The dictionary defines hunger as "the discomfort, pain, or weakness caused by a need for food" or "a desire, need, or appetite for food." If you wait too long to eat, your sensations may intensify until you become ravenous, experiencing what the dictionary describes as "extreme, often frenzied hunger." Beyond this stage, you may become famished, becoming very weak and both physically and mentally impaired.

Remember that the diet industry has taught you that hunger is not meant to have a purpose, and that it should not be acknowledged or taken seriously. You will need to put forth mental energy and concentrate on yourself and your feelings to counter this programming.

One important tip during this stage is to keep some type of food that *you enjoy and find satisfying* handy at all times, as you rediscover your natural hunger cues. Hunger can sometimes be a frightening sensation, and initially it may cause you to reexperience feelings similar to the pain you felt while depriving yourself during a diet or the loss of control you felt when bingeing. Thus it's vital to satisfy your hunger when you become aware of it, so that you will learn to experience hunger as a positive rather than a negative sensation. This will allow you to avoid becoming desperately hungry in situations where no desirable, satiating food choices are available.

Stage Two: Practice Eating Naturally

Eat a meal at one of your favorite restaurants. (A quick note: if you find this idea intimidating, you can do this exercise in your own home; I'll explain how at the end of this section.) It doesn't matter whether you pick a fast-food place or a fancy restaurant; what matters is that you enjoy the food there. Take along a journal, so you can record your experiences—or, if you prefer, take along a trusted friend with whom you can share your feelings.

Plan to arrive at the restaurant slightly hungry but not famished. If you have difficulty identifying your hunger, eat a small snack and then wait at least three hours before you go to the restaurant.

At the restaurant, instead of ordering a "legal" food, open the menu and select any (and I mean *any*) entrée that sounds good to you. As you consider your selection, write yourself an affirming note—for instance, "I am going to eat whatever I desire on this menu, because I am hungry. When I begin to feel full, I will slow down and pay attention to my body. When I become full, it will be OK to stop, because I know that the next time I am hungry, I can again eat whatever I want." Give yourself permission to order *anything you desire* and order a good-sized portion of food—no diet plates or small servings.

When your food arrives, savor it, concentrating on the pleasurable feelings you experience as you eat. When you're about halfway through your meal, stop for a few minutes and have a few sips of water while you write down your feelings in your journal or talk them over with your friend. Notice how you feel after eating the foods you desire. Do you feel slightly anxious or guilty? Are you excited or experiencing a sense of freedom? There is no "right" or "wrong" feeling; what is important is to get in touch with your physical and emotional responses as you eat.

Before you finish your meal, again take a moment to acknowledge how you are feeling physically. Do you have a "stuffed" feeling inside, or are you experiencing a sense of anxiety or emptiness? Do you have a specific craving? Are you thirsty?

At this time, also decide if you would like to order dessert. Because desserts are highly "charged" foods for dieters, this can be an anxiety-provoking action. If you find yourself worrying about what your waiter or other diners will think if they hear you ordering Mississippi mud cake or apple pie with ice cream, remember that your goal is to accept and respect your hunger—and that this is the biggest step toward diet-free health and fitness. Hold your head high and order assertively, and recognize that your goal is more important than the reactions of a waiter or a nearby diner you don't even know.

When you are done with your meal, pay attention to your body and notice if you feel satiated. (See page 111.) Do you feel full? Did you enjoy the food? Do you really feel that you want more? Write down your feelings in your journal before you leave the restaurant.

Repeat this step four or five times, visiting different restaurants if you like. Eating in restaurants is an excellent way to begin freeing yourself from dieting, because it allows you the freedom to choose foods you like while offering you the "safety net" of being in a restaurant with a limited amount of food on your plate.

If you are uncomfortable with the idea of partaking in this experience in a restaurant, however, you can do this exercise at home. Just ensure that you won't be interrupted, that the television is off, that you are eating foods you truly desire, and that you are fully committed to concentrating on yourself. As in the restaurant activity, it's crucial to write in your journal or talk to a friend so that you reflect on your experience and concentrate on your feelings.

Stage Three: Buy and Enjoy the Foods You Like

Once you feel comfortable eating your favorite foods in a restaurant, you are ready to begin bringing these foods into your own home.

Again, pick a time when you're not hungry. Go to your favorite grocery store, take a cart, and go slowly up and down each aisle. Pick out the foods you want to eat for the next few days—not foods you "should" eat but foods you crave. Pick Doritos for dinner, frozen pizza for breakfast, or cinnamon rolls for lunch if you want. Remember that *there are no good or bad foods*. If you long for it, buy it.

Take the food home and—this is the most important part—eat it whenever you want, but only if and when you feel hungry. To eat naturally, you'll need to break the habit of eating at the "right" times and instead learn to be patient and wait until it's the right time for your body—that is, when you're really hungry. When you do sense that you're hungry, be careful not to allow your hunger to continue for a long time without eating.

When you first start eating any foods you desire, as I've noted, you may consume huge amounts of high-fat, sugary, or high-calorie foods. (One of my friends bought boxes of brownie mix and ate them raw, mixing them with Eggbeaters so she wouldn't get salmonella.) This is part of the cure for the disease of dieting, so do not be self-critical if you think you've eaten "too much" food. In fact, tell yourself, "I can eat this food *whenever* I'm hungry, tomorrow, and next week if I want." Allow yourself to eat any food you want, simply *because you're hungry and you want it*, and reassure yourself that the food will be there again for you when you're hungry again. Also reassure yourself that you will note and respect your feelings of satiation as you increasingly learn to identify these sensations.

As you learn to eat naturally, focus on enjoying your meals. If you enjoy cooking, take the time to plan and prepare wonderful meals for yourself. If not, order out Chinese food, pizza, or any other foods you enjoy. During this time, try not to deprive yourself of any food you desire. If you crave a Taco Bell burrito, get one instead of trying to satisfy yourself with a tuna sandwich. If you find yourself longing for chocolate ice cream, but all you have is low-fat frozen yogurt from your dieting days, drive to the store and buy the real thing. Treat yourself as you would treat an honored guest and try to satisfy your every whim.

Even though I'm never tempted to binge anymore, I do sometimes overeat. Usually it's because I've come home hungry and denied that hunger, telling myself, "There's no time to eat—I have too much to do." The result: I find myself, an hour later, grazing on any food that comes to hand. I know that I'd be better off slowing down and making myself a nice sandwich, rather than letting my hunger get out of control.

If you spot the same pattern in your life, make planning and preparing your meals an important part of your day. Take the time to make something appealing, no matter how rushed you are, and remember that your need for a nice meal is as important as any of the jobs on your to-do list.

Continue to go to the store every few days, buying any foods that sound satisfying to you. Pay attention to the types of food you're hungry for. Do you want something salty? Sweet? Smooth? Savory? Begin to sense the signals your body is sending and analyze how you feel when you are hungry, when you eat, and after you eat. In particular, pay attention to the emotions and physical sensations you feel after you've gone for several hours without eating. Hunger means different things to different people, so notice if you feel dizziness, headaches, cravings, anxiety, weakness, a growling or "empty" stomach, or other sensations. Also, note the physical and emotional sensations you feel when you've eaten enough.

In addition, continue to pay attention to emotional triggers that make you want to eat. If you keep a journal, list the triggers you identify. (For additional ideas on identifying your triggers, see Chapter 14.) If you discover that you always eat when your mother criticizes you, or when you're bored or stressed, or at specific times of day, explore your feelings at these times. As I noted earlier, we often use food as a replacement for unmet needs or as a means of subduing emotions we are afraid to confront. Facing these needs and feelings, rather than denying them, can lead you to solutions that will reduce your urge to eat when you're not hungry.

Sarah, thirty-eight years old, grew up with a very overweight mother and sister. Her family ate dinner together every night, paying little attention to calorie counting or nutrition. Sarah's mother proudly served large family meals, and dinner was a time when the family came together and shared in the pleasure of the feast and the security and safety that family meals represented.

As Sarah reached puberty, she began to gain weight, and by fourteen she was known as the "chubby" girl on the block. On the surface Sarah never seemed bothered by her weight. Being big was a part of her family's identity, and Sarah saw herself as destined to a life of obesity. "I don't mind calling myself fat," she said during a therapy session. "I like myself anyway, and I'm not going to diet. I'm just one of those fat girls."

Sarah didn't have an eating disorder, and she didn't suffer from low self-esteem. However, she worried that her obesity could cause health problems, and deep down she felt that if she lost weight she would feel more attractive and be less self-conscious. As we explored her eating pattern, she acknowledged that she "ate on the go," with little awareness of whether or not she was hungry or satiated. She ate a full-course dinner just about every night, and if she didn't have time to cook, she'd stop at Burger King on the way home and pick up a Whopper with cheese, super-sized fries, a vanilla milk shake, and an apple pie. She also loved curling up in front of the TV after dinner with a big bag of Doritos and a bottle of Sprite. Breakfast was pancakes or a stop at McDonald's for an Egg McMuffin and hash browns.

Gradually Sarah realized that she ate for comfort, security, and to occupy her time. Coming from a family that placed huge emotional value on food, she ate big meals, with almost no awareness of the sensations of hunger and satiation, because of the emotional responses to food that she'd learned as a child.

Sarah had no trouble eating the foods she desired, but she found the concentration exercise far more challenging. As she did the exercise daily, and increasingly became aware of her body's physical sensations, she began to realize that she could actually lose weight simply by respecting her body's signals. She also learned to acknowledge her emotional needs (see Step Three), and took up a gentle exercise program that fit her busy lifestyle (see Step Five). Gradually Sarah lost weight, and while she recognizes that she'll never be model thin—an unrealistic and unhealthy goal, given her genetic heritage—she also realizes that she doesn't have to be "one of those fat girls" either.

As you learn to experience and trust your hunger, your friends and family may be surprised at your new eating patterns—whether it appears to them that you are eating more or (as Sarah did) eating less. This may be a good opportunity for you to talk with them about how dieting has harmed you and what you are doing to free yourself from food preoccupations. (Be sure you read Step Eight, "Break Through the Secrecy," in preparation for sharing your thoughts and feelings with others.) It's also a good idea to have your friends and family members read this book so they too will understand that you are following the path toward obtaining a healthy, attractive body and developing a relaxed relationship with food.

The Healing Process

Eventually, as you give yourself permission to experience and enjoy hunger, you will notice remarkable changes. First you will start to recognize which foods you really desire, and you will probably be surprised to discover that as you begin to identify and then eat the foods you actually want to eat, you will experience a sense of satisfaction during meals. As guilt fades, so too will

Own What You Eat—and Notice Yourself

As you allow yourself to eat the foods you want, learn to "own what you eat." This means taking the time to experience and enjoy the food you eat, the opposite of what happens when you graze or binge.

Also, *notice yourself* when you eat. Pay attention to how you feel before, during, and after a meal and identify your hunger and your satiation. Make a conscious choice to notice yourself when you begin to graze, binge, or engage in non-hunger-based eating and to pause (even if for just a moment) to become aware of your feelings and sensations. As you do this, it is critical to remind yourself that the food you're eating will be perfectly fine to eat, and much more enjoyable to eat, if you choose to wait, be patient, and eat when you feel physically hungry.

In addition to paying attention to your feelings when you eat, notice yourself when you are getting hungry and take the necessary time to sit down and eat the foods you really want.

> Julie, one of my patients, says, "Some nights my husband gets home late. I've discovered that if I wait that long to eat dinner, I'm likely to start grazing out of hunger. Now I pay attention to my body's messages, and if I find myself 'zoning out' and eating handfuls of chips or crackers, I remind myself, 'You'll enjoy yourself more if you take the time to decide what you really want for dinner and make it now.'"

As you free yourself from dieting, realize that freedom and responsibility are interconnected. You have the freedom to eat whatever you want, whenever you want, but with that freedom comes the responsibility of identifying your needs and your hunger and satiation, recognizing and acknowledging your feelings when you eat, and fully experiencing the act of eating.

This is particularly important if you binge or graze, either for emotional reasons or because you've developed the habit of eating just for the sake of eating. When you make eating a conscious act, you'll be far less likely to "zone out" and eat food you don't even want.

the sense of being disconnected when you eat. In addition, your sense of anxiety at the end of a meal—a common reaction among dieters accustomed to telling themselves after a too-small meal, "I'm still hungry, but I can't eat any more"—will fade. You will begin to feel full and satisfied after eating normal amounts of food. Gradually, as you continue to allow yourself the freedom to eat freely, you will discover that food no longer holds you in thrall and that you can eat when you want and stop when you want.

These changes won't happen overnight or even in a few weeks. Avoid setting arbitrary goals, and don't worry if you go for weeks or months without a binge and then overeat on several occasions. (This is especially likely to happen if you experience an emotional upset.) Consider any binges not as a setback but as part of your healing process. If you do binge, instead of beating yourself up and condemning yourself for your failures, use the binge as a learning opportunity. Find some time to be alone and analyze what occurred. What triggers led to the binge? Was it hunger that went unsatisfied too long or anxiety, boredom, or loneliness? At what point during the binge did you feel you lost control? Did you remind yourself during the episode that you would be hungry again another time and that when you did become hungry it would be OK to eat the foods you desire whenever you wanted?

Realize that every dieter going through this step does at some time experience a binge or eats for reasons other than hunger. It is through complete self-acceptance, self-understanding, and kindness directed toward our delicate selves that we heal, not by allowing guilt and self-denial to sabotage our healing process. Moreover, there is no logical reason to feel guilty or weak if you binge, because your temporary overeating is merely a lingering symptom of the disease of dieting.

People dying of thirst will, if they find water, drink until they become ill. Similarly, drowning people whose bodies are starved for air will gasp convulsively, desperate to fill their bodies with oxygen. Like them, you are suffering the physical and emotional effects of chronic deprivation, and your body's initial response is to crave food desperately. When you fully realize that you can eat whenever and whatever you please when you become hungry, and that you will be able to—and want to—stop eating when you feel satiated, food will hold no more emotional control over you than the air you breathe or the water you drink.

It's difficult to believe this at first, because diet books tell you that your impulses and desires are self-destructive and that you cannot be trusted. But they are wrong: it is *dieting itself* that transforms your impulses and desires into destructive forces, by artificially caging and denying them, and it is only by taking your needs and desires seriously that you will achieve true fitness. Taking yourself seriously means respecting your body when it feels hungry, listening to your body when it tells you that you are full or satiated, and eating the foods that you desire. It is only by taking this great leap of faith, and accepting the validity of your hunger and your ability to respond to it, that you can break the pattern of starving and overeating.

What About Nutrition?

If you've never paid attention to the nutritional content of what you eat, you may find—once you gain the ability to sense hunger and satiation, and you give yourself permission to eat any food at any time when you're actually hungry—that it's helpful to educate yourself about nutrition.

If you do so, however, be sure not to make lists of "good" and "bad" foods. In fact, as you do learn about nutrition, you'll be surprised to learn that many of the foods you've considered "bad" are foods that do wonderful things for your body. For instance, canola oil—one of those "evil" fats you've been taught to avoid—is rich in omega-3 fatty acids, which can help keep your brain, eyes, heart, and other organs healthy. (Omega-3 fatty acids are particularly crucial for early brain development, which is another reason that putting very young children on diets can be dangerous.) Olive oil, too, can be healthy for your heart and your mental health. And believe it or not, chocolate is now gaining scientific praise because it's packed with particular cell-protecting antioxidants!

The more you learn about the foods that keep your body healthy, the more you'll be interested in eating them. But this time if you select a salad or an apple, it will be because you *want* it, not to conform to externally driven eat-

What Does Satiation Feel Like?

The dictionary definition of satiation is "to satisfy to the full; gratify completely—being filled so full that all pleasure or desire is lost." Here's how my patients define their sense of satiation:

- "I feel pleasantly full and I recognize that if I keep eating, it probably won't feel good."
- "I tell myself to slow down because I know if I continue to eat, I won't feel comfortable."
- "Based on what I've learned in therapy, I concentrate on myself and remind myself that I'm free to have the good food later on when I'm hungry again."
- "I feel a sense of well-being, and the anxiety I felt when I was hungry goes away."

If you eat to the point of feeling bloated, exhausted, or to the point your clothes become noticeably tighter, you've probably eaten past the point of satiation. At first it may be difficult to identify your body's satiation signals. Just as we've been taught to ignore the sensation of hunger, we've forgotten what being "full" feels like, and don't trust our own experience of satiation. Relearning this skill requires a concentrated effort.

ing guidelines that leave you feeling chronically dissatisfied. You'll be amazed at how much more tempting a cantaloupe is when you eat it by choice and not because a diet plan orders you to.

The process of learning to trust your hunger takes time and patience, particularly if you've dieted for many years. How will you know when you've truly recovered from food preoccupations? You'll find yourself leaving the last piece of pizza in the box not because you can't have it but because *you don't want it.* You'll eat a scoop of ice cream for dessert after a nice dinner and feel full. You'll lick the spoon when you frost a cake, but you won't feel tempted to eat half the cake. You'll eat one or two chocolate chip cookies without feeling guilty and without the desperate urge to finish the entire plateful of cookies. And you'll enjoy healthy foods more than ever, because you'll eat them by choice.

When you reach this goal, you will have the tools you need to achieve and maintain your personal ideal weight. With your body dictating how much food you desire, and diet-induced bingeing no longer sabotaging your efforts, your calorie intake will adjust to your calorie expenditure. With time, the extra pounds will melt off, as your body no longer lowers its metabolism in response to recurrent episodes of starvation—the very mechanisms that made you gain weight when you dieted.

As you learn to eat without dieting, you will rediscover the relaxed, joyous relationship with food that you enjoyed as a child. You will no longer feel afraid to have food in your home, to order what you want from a menu, or to enjoy an ice cream cone on a hot day. Using your newfound ability to *notice* yourself and heed your body's messages when you eat, you'll be able to recognize non-hunger-based eating and realize that you can wait to eat until you're truly hungry. You'll be able to indulge in any food you love without worrying about losing control—and as you free yourself from yo-yo diets and chronic weight cycling, you will attain the fit, beautiful body that is your birthright.

Step Five: Straight Talk About Exercise

"I wish it were common knowledge that exercise shouldn't hurt, defeat, bore, or burden you."

Fitness expert Joan Price[1]

My heart races, and my feet pound the ground. I'm six years old, playing tag with friends, the wind ruffling my hair as I run as fast as I can. We're laughing, breathless, hoping the game will never end. I collapse, giggling, as a friend catches me and yells, "Tag!"

Flash forward twenty years. Feet pounding, heart racing, I run through the park, mile after mile. But I'm not enjoying this run. If the wind is blowing, I don't notice it. Instead I count the miles I run, measuring them against the calories I ate earlier when I broke my diet and binged on home-baked muffins.

My stomach aches, but I can't stop. I can't stop until I burn the calories, undo the damage, and atone for my loss of control.

THINK BACK TO your elementary school days. Do you remember the thrill of riding a bike by yourself for the first time or flying down the sidewalk on a skateboard? Do you remember racing home against the rain or playing jump rope games at recess or dancing the Hokey Pokey?

In those days you knew a simple truth: moving is fun. Our bodies crave movement, just as they crave food, air, and sunlight. Children instinctively love to use their bodies—to jump, run, twist, turn, leap, and dance. To a child, moving means freedom and joy, good health and strength.

Now think about how adults feel about exercise. When we talk about it, we talk about how many miles we need to run, how many calories we should burn off, how much punishment we need to endure to make up for enjoying a bagel or a steak. We carefully tape charts to our refrigerators, listing the calories we expend in a half hour of running or an hour of aerobics. We say to ourselves:

"I'm so tired . . . but I should go to the gym or I'll gain back the pound I lost."
"I'm so ashamed . . . I haven't exercised in days. I'll need to do a harder workout today."
"I feel so guilty . . . I ate so much last night, I'll need to jog at least a mile."
"I'm so embarrassed . . . I can't let anyone see how much weight I've gained. I'll need to do an hour of aerobics every night until my thighs aren't so ugly."

We think of these self-flagellating exercise routines, mistakenly, as discipline. Exercise indeed requires discipline and a serious commitment to our own well-being. But as psychologist Erich Fromm notes,

How does one practice discipline? It is essential . . . that discipline should not be practiced like a rule imposed on oneself from the outside, but that it becomes an expression of one's own will; that it is felt as pleasant, and that one slowly accustoms oneself to a kind of behavior which one would eventually miss if one stopped practicing it. It is one of the unfortunate aspects of our Western concept of discipline that its practice is supposed to be somewhat painful and only if it is painful can it be good. The East has recognized long ago that that which is good for man—for his body and for his soul—must also be agreeable.[2]

Discipline is a form of loving ourselves, respecting ourselves, and taking our bodies and ourselves seriously. When we see the discipline of exercise in this light, we undertake it joyously as a commitment to giving our bodies what they need. But when we equate discipline with punishment, we turn a willing commitment into a sentence. What is the message we send ourselves? That we are weak and bad and that exercise is penance for our sin of eating. That exercise is grueling and painful and boring. That exercise is something we "should do" or "must do," never something we do for the sheer joy of it.

As a result, some of us become driven, compulsive exercisers—a phenomenon the medical community now recognizes as "exercise bulimia"— and cause permanent damage to our bodies. Far more of us, discouraged by our failure to stick with impossibly difficult exercise routines, give up altogether, because we see no realistic alternative to a sedentary lifestyle.

Maria hadn't exercised for years when I first met her and didn't view herself as athletic or capable of engaging in a meaningful exercise routine. That's because, at 5'4" and two hundred pounds, she believed she'd already lost the battle. "I'm destined to be fat," she told me. "And it's my fault, because I can't stick with the exercise programs my doctor recommends. I just can't do it." But Maria needed to exercise, because type II diabetes, the type that often strikes overweight adults who don't exercise, ran in her family.

For Maria the stakes were high. She knew that she needed to exercise for life—but she feared setting herself up for another failure, more guilt, and more pain.

When we think of exercise as punishment, or believe that we must exercise even when we don't want to, we cheat ourselves out of the joy of physical movement. We stop viewing our bodies as potential sources of pleasure, to be nurtured and treated gently and with dignity, and begin to view them as enemies that we must fight.

When we do this, we stop dancing for pleasure or running for the simple joy of running. Instead we develop grueling exercises to burn off calories, remove cellulite, and punish ourselves for eating. We replace our bikes with Exercycles that calculate miles ridden and calories burned. We replace leisurely walks with treadmills, so we can exercise faster and harder and more relentlessly. In the process we build yet another wall between ourselves and the pleasures that make us human.

Ironically, this sacrifice may lead us farther away from health and slimness. Many of us, like Maria, simply give up on exercise programs that require too much pain and too much time. Others feel like failures if they don't exercise to the point of exhaustion at least once a day. I can remember my days in medical school, when I watched perfectionist friends desperately trying to work off calories by jogging for miles, combining their runs with one or two aerobic classes a day.

I too followed a rigid exercise schedule, until my mind and body rebelled one day and I decided, "No more!" I felt a tremendous relief when I stopped—and even greater relief when I didn't turn into the obese person I was running from. Luckily, I'd begun learning by then to trust my body, and I didn't react by abandoning exercise altogether, as Maria did. Instead I came to my senses and adopted the same strategy for exercise as I had for eating: I began exercising when I felt like it and engaging in physical activities that gave me joy.

And guess what? It worked. I remember the amazement of my friends, who were still torturing themselves on a daily basis, when they realized that I could be fit without following a grueling exercise regimen.

In fact, when I abandoned my tortuous exercise program and discovered my own natural "exercise cycle," the pattern of exercise that fit my needs and lifestyle, I actually became more fit. That's because I learned to listen to my body. For instance, in the summer, I love to exercise, but in the winter I tend to be a homebody, snuggled up on the couch with a book. Because the winters are cold where I live, this makes perfectly good sense, so I accept it. I keep in shape with light and fun indoor exercises, but I don't drive myself to despair by telling myself, "Shame on you! You're a bad person for not jogging five miles today." And I don't force myself to perform grueling exercise routines that I'd most likely just abandon, leaving me feeling guilty and frustrated.

Conversely, I discovered that in the summertime I tended to push myself hard when I exercised and frequently wound up with injuries as a result. Once I identified my overcompetitive pattern, I learned not to "raise the bar" every time I ran, and instead to let my body set its natural pace. When I do, my body is healthier, I suffer fewer injuries, and I spend less time recovering from self-inflicted wounds.

My current fitness plan is far less demanding than the hard-core, five-miles-a-day, four-days-a-week routine I once followed, but it works far better. I couldn't keep up that rigorous, no-fun routine, and I felt a tremendous burden of guilt each time I gave up . . . which led to more bingeing, more guilt, more weight gain, and a lower level of fitness.

Yet the workout I followed was exactly what most fitness gurus recommend. "Hardbody" workouts are in, and exercise experts no longer suggest, "Play tag with your children" or "Turn on the radio and dance to your favorite songs." Instead they tell us to exercise to the point of pain. More reps. Add weights. Cross-train. Hire a personal trainer. Make it burn. Make it hurt.

What they're not telling us is that all of this pain and sacrifice often leads to failure. Yet year after year, we're told to sacrifice our time and our bodies to excruciating exercise, just as we sacrifice our physical and mental health to dieting. Many men and women, like Maria, simply say "I quit" and stop exercising altogether.

Hardbody workouts are virtually impossible for people who aren't natural athletes, and the very individuals who need exercise most often give up and become sedentary, believing that—as Maria told me— "exercise is for other people." As a result, many develop diabetes (now reaching epidemic proportions in America) or put themselves at risk for obesity, heart disease, and even some forms of cancer.

The tragedy is that none of this is necessary.

The Big Lie: "No Pain, No Gain"

In her therapy sessions, Maria and I talked for hours about her weight, her fears about diabetes, and her life. I learned about her abusive, very obese mother, her alcoholic, unavailable father, and the tremendous inner strength that helped her survive her childhood. I knew that this inner strength would help her over-

come her belief that she was doomed to develop diabetes and to face the reality that her life depended on getting fit.

Clearly, however, the standard advice of today's fitness gurus—"Put in an hour at the gym every day!" "Exercise until it hurts!"—made no sense in Maria's world. She worked long days as a nurse's aide, caring for sick relatives in her "spare" time. She had little money and no time to nurture her own needs, and the last thing she needed was more pain or sacrifice in her life.

It's a given: movement can help keep your body fit and beautiful. In fact, obesity expert Kelly Brownell says, "Whether participants in weight control programs are exercising is the single strongest correlate of the long-term maintenance of weight loss." More important, movement facilitates mental well-being, and it's easier to achieve any goal—including fitness—if you feel good. But trainers who say that fitness and well-being require suffering are simply wrong, and scientific research proves it.

A new Dutch study, for instance, used portable motion sensors to study the activities of thirty adults between the ages of twenty-two and thirty-two. The result: *exercising moderately (for instance, by doing housework, gardening, and walking) throughout the day burned more energy than did bursts of high-impact activities.* In addition, the researchers say, participants were far more willing to participate in moderate activity than in grueling workouts.[3] In other words, moderate, enjoyable exercise takes pounds off more effectively over the long term than punishing regimens, and it's more likely to provide lasting benefits because you're more likely to stick with it.

But what about other health benefits—a stronger heart, a reduced risk of diabetes, and so on? Again, the "experts" who say that exercise only helps if it hurts are wrong. For instance:

- A study of nearly forty thousand female health professionals, forty-five years of age or older, found that one hour of walking per week significantly reduces the risk of coronary heart disease. [4]
- Researchers in Japan report that walking twenty or more minutes a day can lower blood pressure significantly. [5]
- An hour a day of moderate exercise dramatically reduces the risk of diabetes, even if the activity is split into several sessions—for

instance, thirty minutes of housecleaning during the day, and thirty minutes of walking in the evening.[6]

In short, there's no reason to punish your body physically if you want to lose weight and stay fit. Moderate exercise, three to five times a week, will help protect your heart, lower your blood pressure, and help prevent diabetes—and it can trim inches off your figure as well.

In fact Brownell believes, based on research data, that the weight loss associated with exercise stems more from improved self-esteem than from energy expenditure. Fun, healthy exercise makes us feel good about ourselves, and feeling good translates into fewer episodes of emotional grazing or bingeing. Exercise also improves our mood, because it produces "feel good" chemicals called *endorphins*. Exercise helps us maintain our concentration on our physical and emotional state and on ourselves. More and more research shows, too, that reducing your stress by exercising can help you lose weight by lowering your levels of a hormone called *cortisol*, which is elevated in people experiencing stress and is associated with weight gain (see Step Seven). And as we discover that moving our bodies can be a pleasurable activity, rather than a grueling obsession or a punitive response to eating, we begin to move more and more, for the simple joy of it.

Suffering and pain aren't what we need from an exercise program. We need, instead, to return to the wisdom of our childhood, when we used our bodies freely and happily and moved to the beat of our inner urges. And in an age when each of us is stressed, pressured, overworked, and pulled in competing directions by multiple responsibilities, we need exercise opportunities that will nurture our souls and make our lives happier—not add to our stress or make us feel inadequate.

Maria and I designed an exercise plan tailor-made to help her become fit, healthy, and trim without subjecting her to stressful demands on her time, energy, or finances. She started simply, by adding a fifteen-minute walk to her daily routine, twice a week. In addition, she made weekly visits to a good friend who was training to be a massage therapist. Massages allowed Maria to get in touch with her body and feel positive about her physicality, while she refreshed herself spiritually by talking with someone supportive and fun.

Over the next two years Maria continued exercising, gradually adding to her activities as she discovered that she enjoyed walking, dancing, and other physical activities. Now she works out an average of four times a week, taking long walks and even participating in a beginning dance class for adults. She doesn't "stress out" over exercising, because she knows she can take a few days off without feeling guilty—but she finds that if she misses a week or so she actually craves physical activity. How well is Maria's fun and easy exercise program working? She's lost more than fifty pounds!

The Self-Fulfilling Prophecy

In part because of her experiences as a chubby child, Maria pictured herself as a nonathlete, a self-image with potentially devastating health consequences. Always picked last for the softball team, and considered "too fat" for dance or gymnastics, Maria internalized the idea that fitness was beyond her reach.

My friend Bob, in contrast, has a strong image of himself as athletic, in part because of his earlier experience as a pro basketball player. Even today, when his life is filled with the responsibilities of a career and fatherhood, he instinctively sees himself as an athlete and considers exercise as much a part of his day as taking a shower. He hits the gym almost daily, not because he's obsessed with sculpting his body or losing weight but simply because he loves exercise. (He exercises when and how he wants; some days he works out hard, and others he simply relaxes in the sauna, knowing that he can take a day or two off without getting out of shape and comfortable in the awareness that relaxing his muscles and mind is a part of his overall fitness and well-being.)

From an early age, Maria viewed herself as unfit and Bob viewed himself as fit. In part, of course, both self-images are based on reality; it's unlikely that Maria, under any circumstances, would have become an Olympic athlete or a professional ballplayer. But society's expectations, and their views of themselves, also helped shape Bob's love of exercise and Maria's sedentary lifestyle.

One of the most powerful phenomena in psychology is the self-fulfilling prophecy, which means that our preconceived ideas can alter our futures. When a boisterous little boy hears his teacher say that he's bad, he tends to fulfill that prophecy by increasing his "acting out" behavior. The same is true

When Exercise Hurts

She arrives at the gym too early and stays too late. . . . There's a look in her eye: both glazed and frantic. She's the one in the back of the aerobics class who, during the cool-down, frenetically jogs in place while everyone else stretches languorously. She will not get off that bike (that treadmill, that track, that rower) until she has hit the desired time. 28:35 is not good enough, ever. 28:35 is failure. 30:00 is completion, no excuses.

Elizabeth Krieger, "Confessions of a Stair Mistress," in Salon,
January 4, 1999

In a society that values stick-thin "hardbodies," our relationship with exercise is as distorted as our relationship with food. Just as we starve ourselves when our bodies cry out for food, we exercise when our bodies need rest, sleep, or pampering. (Have you ever exercised when you were sick? Exercised when you were already exhausted, to work off a doughnut? Run in spite of sore knees or shinsplints?) We do exercises we don't enjoy, in artificial routines that bear no relation to what our bodies need or our spirit craves.

Worse yet, in our quest to become ever harder and leaner, we often damage our bodies seriously and permanently. Large numbers of young women, in particular, subject their bodies to grueling exercise regimens that alter their hormone levels, stop their menstrual cycles (a condition called *amenorrhea*), and cause severe bone loss, putting them at risk for osteoporosis by the time they're forty. The pattern of eating disorders, excess exercise, and amenorrhea, known by the medical community as "the Female Athlete Triad," affects tens of thousands of young women who are active in sports—a healthy interest that, in their cases, becomes an unhealthy obsession.

(continued)

Intense exercise can also permanently damage men's and women's joints, reduce immune system functioning, deplete the body's stores of disease-fighting antioxidants, and cause serious anemia. In addition it can break down muscle fibers faster than they can recover, actually making it harder to become truly fit.

Moreover, increasing numbers of men and women are crossing the line from strenuous exercise into exercise addiction—a form of addiction almost as dangerous to mental health as alcoholism or drug abuse. "What starts for health and fitness purposes ultimately flips around and begins to control you," says physical education professor Michael Sachs. Men and women who become exercise addicts often abandon relationships and outside interests to train obsessively, exercising even when they have stress fractures or illnesses. According to a recent U.K. study, nearly one in five females who are active athletically show signs of exercise addiction.

of our attitudes about exercise: our beliefs about our own athletic ability and the beliefs of others around us play a powerful role in making us fit or unfit.

Maria's early experiences shaped the negative self-image that she was too clumsy and too "big" for physical activity. Bob's early experiences, in contrast, gave him confidence in his athletic ability. As a result Maria avoided physical movement, becoming even less fit and less athletic and fulfilling the prophecy. Bob, in contrast, honed his skills and transformed his athletic potential into professional-level talent—again, living up to his self-image and the image others had of him.

If you're having difficulty finding or sticking with an exercise program, a negative self-image may be holding you back. Changing that self-image is not an easy task; thus it's important to begin with an exercise plan that doesn't violate your current view of your own athleticism. (For instance, Maria began with simple walking, discovered that she enjoyed it, and is now branching out into dance and other activities. If she'd started by trying to run a marathon, she probably would have given up and reinforced her initial self-image as a nonexerciser.) It's also important to select a program that matches your current level of fitness, so you won't injure yourself or become discouraged.

So start from where you are now—but as you begin to enjoy exercising, don't be limited by preconceived ideas about what you should or shouldn't try and what you can and can't do. For years I believed that I was "too tall" for ballet. Now I take adult ballet classes, and I love it. These days, however, I'm not concentrating so much on how I look during the class but on how I feel and how I enjoy the atmosphere, the stretching, and the focus on moving my body in unity with the music. Similarly, as you take a leap of faith and allow yourself to participate in activities that give you pleasure, without counting the calories you expend, calculating the heart rate you reach, or focusing on how you look while you're exercising, you're likely to find that your self-image ("I'm

Are You Addicted to Exercise?

"Exercise addiction" is dangerous, both mentally and physically, and sometimes goes hand-in-hand with eating disorders. If you find your-self falling into a pattern of compulsive exercising, be aware of the serious nature of this problem and consider talking with a therapist. Signs of unhealthy exercise obsession include the following.

- You turn down dates or miss activities with friends or family to keep up your exercise schedule.
- You exercise even if you are ill or injured.
- You push yourself to exercise at your maximum capacity almost every day.
- You feel upset and anxious if you miss a workout.
- You feel anxious when you relax, because you feel that you're not burning enough calories.
- You calculate the amount of exercise you need each day to burn off the calories you eat.
- You believe that you will gain weight if you miss even a single day of exercise.

too uncoordinated for tennis/too old to learn to swim/too big to exercise at a public gym") begins to change and that you're capable of enjoying a wide range of activities that you once considered off-limits.

Use the questionnaire that follows to select activities that meet your current fitness attitudes, needs, and abilities. As you try these activities, however, also keep an open mind about experimenting with new ways of moving. Don't feel that you need to limit yourself to aerobics, weight lifting, or other standard forms of exercise; be creative and you may discover that you fall in love with ballroom dancing, martial arts, tai chi, football, yoga, ice skating, or kayaking. Above all, banish the idea that you "must" or "should" exercise and learn to move for the sheer joy of it. When you do, you'll transform exercise from a painful and stressful obligation into a life-affirming, joyous, fitness-enhancing act.

"Where Have You Been/ Where Are You Now?" An Exercise Questionnaire

Instructions

Respond to each of the following phrases with "yes" or "no." Answer "yes" if the phrase sounds like you most of the time. Answer "no" if the phrase does not apply to you most of the time. Remember that "most of the time" means 50 percent or more of the time.

1. I am the athletic type. ☐ Yes ☐ No

2. During my childhood, exercise was part of our family routine. ☐ Yes ☐ No

3. I am physically strong. ☐ Yes ☐ No

4. I participate in a regular exercise regimen. ☐ Yes ☐ No

5. I feel comfortable in a gym or when participating in athletic activities. ☐ Yes ☐ No

6. I am coordinated and agile. ☐ Yes ☐ No

7. I participated in an athletic activity on a regular basis during my childhood. ☐ Yes ☐ No

8. I would like to become more physically active. ☐ Yes ☐ No

9. Since I'm not really fit, I feel that I have almost no hope of developing a regular exercise routine. ☐ Yes ☐ No

10. I feel that I must work out to a level that improves my fitness, even if I feel worse after I exercise. ☐ Yes ☐ No

11. I would be willing to exercise on a regular basis, but only for the purpose of losing weight. ☐ Yes ☐ No

12. Once I plan out my week, I generally stick to my schedule. ☐ Yes ☐ No

13. I consider myself a sedentary person. ☐ Yes ☐ No

14. Once I decide that something is important to me, I do what it takes to make it happen. ☐ Yes ☐ No

15. I would like to participate in a regular exercise plan, but I'm too overweight. ☐ Yes ☐ No

16. I enjoy leaving my house to go to the gym or to work out. ☐ Yes ☐ No

17. One or both of my parents was physically fit. ☐ Yes ☐ No

18. People like me just don't work out; I'm just not the type. ☐ Yes ☐ No

19. I don't like to exercise, and I will never participate in regular exercise. ☐ Yes ☐ No

20. I believe that once you become an adult, it's not really possible to change in any significant way. ☐ Yes ☐ No

Scoring: Give yourself points as follows:

1. 5 points if yes   _____
2. 2 points if yes   _____
3. 3 points if yes   _____
4. 5 points if yes   _____
5. 5 points if yes   _____
6. 4 points if yes   _____
7. 4 points if yes   _____
8. 4 points if yes   _____
9. 4 points if no   _____
10. 3 points if no   _____
11. 2 points if no   _____
12. 4 points if yes   _____
13. 5 points if no   _____
14. 5 points if yes   _____
15. 4 points if no   _____
16. 4 points if yes   _____
17. 2 points if yes   _____
18. 5 points if no   _____
19. 5 points if no   _____
20. 5 points if no   _____
    Total Points   _____

Note: Before beginning any exercise program, consult with your physician, particularly if you have any medical condition that could affect your ability to exercise safely.

0–20: You perceive yourself as an "outsider" when it comes to athletic activity, and when you read and hear about exercise programs, you easily become overwhelmed and disillusioned. You may doubt that you could ever actually enjoy exercise, and you've probably never participated in a regular exercise regimen. Given your previous lack of exposure to exercise, you deserve commendation for taking the plunge and completing this questionnaire.

To change your lifestyle, you will need to take a leap of faith. Ask yourself: is your self-image as a nonathlete limiting your ability to develop a healthier lifestyle? Are you ready to free yourself from the constraints of this self-perception? If so, begin with the Level One activities outlined in the next section. Let "easy" and "slow" be your goals and be kind to yourself. Also, remember that a short walk or massage is worthwhile in and of itself, especially if you actually enjoy it!

21–40: Physical activity is not entirely foreign to you, but you may feel odd or uncomfortable when you work out or play sports. You've probably toyed with exercising but haven't been able to sustain a long-term routine. Perhaps you've made efforts to partake in a program or joined a health club, but only with reluctance and perhaps even fear or shame. Chances are you quit early on, after becoming exhausted and frustrated. You may sometimes make plans to take up a new fitness program, but probably only out of a desire to lose weight.

    If you've completed this questionnaire, you're interested in challenging your self-image as a nonexerciser and in making exercise a more important part of your lifestyle. My recommendation: start with the Level Two activities outlined later.

41–60: Your background suggests that you enjoy physical activity. However, because of the demands of daily life, or your belief that exercise must be strenuous or painful to be effective, you may not exercise on a regular basis. Perhaps you've started exercise regimens but pushed yourself too hard and wound up giving up or getting injured. If you are comfortable with your current level of exercise, then continue it—but beware of pushing yourself too hard and suffering exercise burnout. For ideas on exercise activities, see my Level Three recommendations.

61–80: You have a healthy attitude toward exercise. Exercise probably became part of your natural routine in childhood, and you have a positive view of your fitness capability. Continue to make exercise or physical activity an important part of your life while being careful not to fall into the overexercise trap, and you'll be on the right path to taking off excess pounds and keeping them off. See my Level Four recommendations.

Level One Recommendations

Begin by expanding your definition of *exercise*: You don't need to run, sweat, or grunt—*any opportunity to partake in an activity where your mind and body are united* counts as exercise!

If you feel shy or uncomfortable going to a gym, a ten-minute walk, twice weekly, is an excellent first step toward better fitness. In addition, if you enjoy and can afford it, get a regular massage. Consider buying a good beginner's exercise tape, too. (A tip: rent exercise videos from your local library and try them out to see which you enjoy.) One of my favorite activities is gardening, an underrated form of stress reduction and exercise.

Get in touch with your physicality by taking a Jacuzzi or sauna after a cool shower or, if this isn't possible, taking a bubble bath. Afterward, try some gentle stretching (for ideas, I recommend the book *Stretching* by Bob Anderson), perhaps followed by another cooldown shower and Jacuzzi. A facial also is a good way to reconnect your physical and mental being.

If you feel daring, consider karate or a dance class (one of my patients discovered that she loved ballroom dancing) or bowling. Enjoy the activities you pick, but don't make yourself continue with them any longer than you want to; for instance, don't force yourself to bowl three games if you feel like bowling only one. Remember that your goal is to make yourself healthier and fitter by nurturing yourself and reducing your stress level.

Level Two Recommendations

Think about bowling, softball, or any other type of entry-level team activity. Many people who aren't natural-born athletes love team sports, because of the combination of exercise and social interaction. (Mall-walking groups offer the same benefit if you're looking for something less strenuous.)

If group activities aren't for you, start a walking routine, two or three times a week, for fifteen to twenty minutes. If you feel like it, try jogging for a few minutes during each walk. Do a few jumping jacks, sit-ups, or push-ups along with stretches in the morning before work. Jump rope with your kids or buy yourself a Hula Hoop. Take an in-line skating class or start going out dancing occasionally with friends.

Dance, tai chi, and yoga classes are enjoyable, low-stress fitness activities. Also, consider buying several exercise tapes and try out fun activities including biking, swimming, horseback riding, or even a regular game of Frisbee with your dog.

Focus, above all, on giving yourself permission to enjoy your physicality. If you can, start getting regular massages. If you belong to a gym, don't feel that you must engage in a strenuous workout every time you're there; instead, try going occasionally just for the enjoyment of stretching for several minutes and then taking a Jacuzzi, steam, or sauna. When you do, you'll learn to reconnect with your physicality and rediscover your body as a source of pleasure.

Level Three Recommendations

By selecting the right exercise program, you can make your natural athleticism work for you. Avoid falling into hard-core, heavy-duty exercise programs that trim off inches for a little while but may not work in the long run because they can cause exercise burnout. (This mistake is similar to thinking that "quick fix" weight-loss plans will solve your problems.) Find activities that you *enjoy* instead of merely choosing those that burn calories. When you do, you'll achieve excellent long-term results. You probably already know some of the activities that you do and don't like, so select activities that you prefer and drop those that bore or stress you.

For instance, are you starting to dread your usual five-mile run? If so, give yourself permission to take a leisurely bike ride or swim instead. Too tired for a thirty-minute workout? Then exercise for fifteen minutes instead, and see if you feel like continuing. And if you find yourself setting harder and harder goals ("I need to run an eight-minute mile"), reconsider your priorities. Remember that participating in regular, moderate exercise is smarter and more effective than forcing yourself to participate in intense, grueling workouts that can lead to injury or burnout.

Because you like physical activity, you might enjoy the challenge of participating in a run or bike race for charity—a great way to get exercise while meeting new people and helping your community. You might even want to train for a half-marathon, if running is your favorite activity. Just be sure to make fun and stress reduction—not calorie-burning—your top priorities!

Level Four Recommendations

Keep up the good work! Your goal is to establish a healthy and pleasant exercise routine, intermingling challenging activities with peaceful and relaxing mind/body experiences. If you find yourself becoming bored, vary your exercise routine with creative new activities; for instance, if you're tired of jogging every morning, try taking up kickboxing, spin cycling, in-line skating, even a jazz dance class. Spicing up your exercise routine will motivate you to stick with it.

No matter what level of activity is right for you, concentrate on nurturing yourself through exercise. When you do, you'll feel good—and when you feel good, you'll stick with your fitness plan.

Some days that plan might lead you to be the first person at the gym or to sign up for a challenging fitness run. Other days you'll be found at the spa getting a massage or stretching for a few minutes before you take a leisurely walk. It may seem hard to believe, but all of these activities are active ways of achieving true and lasting fitness.

So forget "no pain, no gain," and instead focus on the joy of swimming, walking, skating, belly dancing, or even Jacuzzi-ing your way to better health and a trimmer body. Expand your definition of exercise to include any activities that help you relieve stress and "connect" your mind and body—and make a commitment, based on self-love and self-affirmation, to make exercise a priority in your life. When you do, you'll see your excess pounds and inches come off more quickly and effortlessly.

Step Six: Get Your Doctor on Your Weight-Loss Team

"You can't solve a problem until you know what it is."

Psychiatrist Sydney Walker[1]

THE TEN-STEP No-Diet Fitness Plan removes the roadblocks keeping you from achieving your goal of weight loss and fitness. For some of you, this includes an invisible roadblock: an undetected medical disorder that's causing you to put on pounds and making weight loss a losing battle.

The good news is that many medical disorders that contribute to weight gain are easy to detect, and if you're diagnosed with one of them, there are treatments that can make you healthier and help you shed unwanted pounds. But to persuade your doctor to check you for these medical problems, you'll need to be assertive.

This can take courage if you're overweight. Few of us enjoy getting check-ups, but it's especially daunting if you're struggling with a weight problem, because doctors aren't always knowledgeable or sympathetic about weight issues. Moreover, there's a chance that your doctor will casually dismiss the suggestion that your weight problem could stem from medical conditions and suggest that you're simply "looking for excuses."

If this happens, be persistent, because getting a thorough checkup can make the difference between permanent weight loss and a lifelong struggle with an undetected medical problem that thwarts your weight-loss efforts. Insisting on a complete examination, while it may be a little intimidating, can pay off for the rest of your life.

When I tell patients with weight issues to get a medical exam, many of them respond, "But I have an annual checkup!" However, a doctor doing a quick annual exam can easily miss the leading medical causes of weight gain. Also, in an era of managed care, too many doctors are quick to prescribe diets without evaluating patients for disorders that can affect body size and weight.

So, as part of your weight-loss plan, visit your doctor for a complete physical. This is a case in which a routine eight-minute, temperature-and-blood-pressure-check visit isn't enough, *especially* if:

- you have additional symptoms that could point to a physical disorder
- you have a family history of any medical problems that can cause weight gain
- you have a family history of being overweight that doesn't seem to be related to food intake
- your weight gain doesn't seem to be related to what you eat

When you make an appointment, try to find a doctor who is willing to listen to you. Too often doctors brush patients' weight-related medical problems aside because they're too diet oriented, too prejudiced against people with weight problems, or too pressured by time constraints to check for the diseases that often underlie weight gain. So be prepared: go into your appointment with a list of any symptoms that concern you (see the lists in this chapter) and insist on a full physical examination and laboratory analyses when indicated.

Above all, whether your physician uncovers any medical problems or not, don't be pressured into accepting another low-calorie or low-carbohydrate diet unless there is a compelling health reason for doing so. Your goal is to remove any medical barriers to fitness, not to become trapped in another fruitless cycle of dieting and weight gain. So tell your doctor the following, at the outset of your appointment.

• You don't want a new "diet plan" unless he or she gives you a valid medical reason, other than weight problems, for accepting one. Tell your doctor that you're very interested in losing weight but that the scientific evidence clearly shows that dieting is usually unsuccessful in helping people achieve long-term weight loss. Explain that you no longer want to invest your time and effort in a method with such a low success rate and such a high rate of adverse medical and psychological effects.

• You don't want a "diet drug" unless your circumstances clearly warrant one. If you're dealing with severe, life-threatening obesity, the benefits of temporary diet drug use may outweigh their risks. But diet drugs usually don't work as a long-term fix, and they can have dangerous or even potentially life-threatening side effects, as the recent recall of fen-phen—a "miracle" pill linked to life-threatening heart conditions in many patients—demonstrates.

• You want a thorough checkup to rule out any medical problems that can cause weight gain or make weight loss difficult.

What are some of the weight-related medical disorders your doctor should rule out in a physical exam? While this isn't a medical textbook, I'm going to introduce you to the most common culprits, because the odds are surprisingly high that you, a good friend, or a family member may suffer from one of them.

Sometimes It *Is* Hormones

Insensitive people laugh when a three-hundred-pound man or woman says, "It's my hormones." But it's not a joke: the hormones that control your body can indeed become unbalanced and cause your weight to spiral, no matter how much you exercise and how little you eat. Among the common hormone-associated problems that can lead to weight gain:

Polycystic Ovary Syndrome (PCOS)

As many as 10 percent of women suffer from this problem, and most don't know it. (Many women find out they have PCOS only when they have difficulty getting pregnant, because the disorder can cause infertility.)

Janet called herself a "professional dieter." Sometimes, when she was lucky, she'd take off five or ten pounds by eating nothing but fruits and vegetables. But she always gained back the weight within a month. And no matter how much she exercised, she couldn't get rid of the "spare tire" around her waist.

What Janet didn't know was that her problem didn't stem from too much food or too little exercise. She had polycystic ovary syndrome (PCOS)—a condition her doctor overlooked at each visit, when he patted her on the shoulder and said, condescendingly, "You're still gaining weight—are you sure you're following that diet I gave you?"

Fortunately, Janet found a new doctor. This physician spotted signs and symptoms of PCOS, and sent her to a reproductive endocrinologist, who put her on medications to adjust her hormones and enhance her body's use of insulin (a function that's impaired in PCOS). As a result, for the first time in years, Janet is losing weight rather than gaining it—and treatment is reducing her risk of diabetes, uterine cancer, and other diseases associated with PCOS.

PCOS usually begins in puberty, but it can occur at any age after that. It appears to occur when a condition called *insulin resistance* can cause a woman's levels of testosterone and luteinizing hormone (LH) to become too high, throwing off her menstrual cycle and causing ovulation to occur infrequently or not at all.

Women with PCOS can gain fifty or more pounds in just a few years, even when they eat the same amount as their thin friends. In addition, PCOS can (but not always) cause these symptoms:

irregular periods
facial hair growth
infertility
depression
male pattern baldness
acne

How Do You Find the Right Doctor?

Locating a doctor who's understanding and sympathetic and won't simply tell you to try another diet isn't always easy. Some suggestions:

• Ask your friends for the names of doctors who are good listeners, show respect for their patients, and perform complete physicals rather than rushing through appointments. Also, ask your friends (especially those with weight issues) whether they've had bad experiences with any of the doctors you're considering seeing.

• When you visit a new doctor, ask questions such as: "What are your thoughts on dieting?" "Do you consider blood tests for patients dealing with weight problems?" "Do you have experience in helping patients lose weight?" "Are you comfortable working with patients who are dealing with weight issues through nondiet methods?"

There are no specific right or wrong answers to these questions, but they'll help you gauge a doctor's style and personality. Look for a doctor who's open-minded, willing to learn, respectful rather than condescending, and willing to at least consider the scientific data showing that diets don't work.

If you have any of these symptoms, ask your doctor to check you for PCOS. Doctors can control many symptoms of PCOS with specially tailored nutrition plans, exercise programs, insulin-reducing drugs such as metformin, and sometimes surgery. (Note: this is one case in which specific eating plans may be necessary.) In addition, getting treatment for the insulin resistance that appears to underlie PCOS can dramatically reduce your risk of diabetes and other life-threatening medical problems.

Hypothyroidism

This common disorder occurs when the thyroid, a butterfly-shaped gland in the throat, either produces too few hormones or can't use these hormones effectively.

Around ten million Americans, most of them women, suffer from hypothyroidism, and most of them aren't aware that they have the problem. All they know is that they gain weight easily and often feel tired and "dragged out." (While fewer men than women suffer from hypothyroidism, you're more likely to go undiagnosed if you're male.) Other common symptoms can include:

slow heart rate
dry, coarse skin

The Invisible Epidemic

Americans suffer from an epidemic of undiagnosed hypothyroidism, according to the Thyroid Foundation of America. According to the organization's estimates:

- 7 million women have undetected hypothyroidism
- 1.6 million women have diagnosed hypothyroidism
- 1.6 million men have undetected hypothyroidism
- 100,000 men have diagnosed hypothyroidism

Because so many women in particular go undiagnosed, the American Association of Clinical Endocrinologists recommends that doctors screen all women over the age of forty for hypothyroidism, even if the women have no obvious symptoms. However, many managed care programs consider the test (which costs about $50) too expensive to use routinely, so don't assume that your doctor will request it without your prompting.

infertility in women
increased menstrual flow in women
a feeling of being cold, even in normal or warm temperatures
concentration and memory problems
muscle cramps
depression
husky voice
loss of hair in the outer part of the eyebrow

Because thyroid problems are so common, and so often missed by doctors, it's important to be assertive and ask your doctor to order a thyroid panel. This is especially true if you're over forty, even if you have no symptoms other than difficulty losing weight.

PMS or PDD

Years ago, as a "recovering dieter," I decided to track my binges and see if I could isolate the triggers that made me eat uncontrollably. As I marked my calendar each month, a clear pattern emerged: most of my binges occurred in the ten days before my periods started. What a comfort, to learn that my seemingly out-of-control behavior had a strong biological basis! Now that I'm aware of how PMS affects my cravings and emotions, I'm extra-careful to avoid becoming overly hungry, tired, or stressed during this time of month.

If you believe that PMS is a problem for you, chart your symptoms for three to four months. The most common symptoms you may experience are:

irritability and anger
depression, sadness, crying jags
bingeing, particularly on high-carbohydrate foods
food cravings
fatigue
"out-of-control" behavior
poor concentration and feeling "scattered"
acne
headaches
weight gain
bowel problems

bloating
breast tenderness

Most women with PMS experience symptoms five to seven days before a period, but some have symptoms both before a period and at mid-cycle (just before ovulation). Still others have PMS symptoms that begin at ovulation and last until their periods begin or symptoms that start at ovulation and continue until the end of their periods.

If your PMS is severe, ask your doctor about medical treatments. If it's mild, be aware of your trigger times and realize that you must work extra-hard to treat yourself kindly on those days. If you can, avoid planning stressful or tiring activities during your PMS days, and be sure to eat frequently so you don't become overly hungry and make yourself vulnerable to bingeing. If you crave certain foods (for instance, high-carbohydrate foods), don't forbid yourself from satisfying these cravings! If you do, you're likely to set yourself up for a serious binge.

In addition, schedule time for meditation, exercise, and other activities that can prevent food cravings and ease other symptoms. Also, ask your doctor about taking extra calcium; several large-scale studies link PMS to calcium deficiency and show that calcium supplements can decrease PMS symptoms by up to half. Some women also report that avoiding salt and excess caffeine and alcohol reduces food cravings and other PMS symptoms. Each woman is unique, however, so see what works for you.

Cushing's Syndrome

Each year thousands of men and women develop Cushing's syndrome, a disorder caused by overproduction of a hormone called *cortisol*. If you have Cushing's syndrome, you're likely to gain weight in your upper body, and you may develop a round face and fat deposits around your neck while your arms and legs stay thin. One common symptom is a "buffalo hump" on the back. Other symptoms can include:

fatigue
weakness
high blood pressure
high blood sugar
depression

backache
headache
thirst
increased urination
impotence in males
cessation of periods in females

Doctors usually spot clear-cut cases of this disorder, but when symptoms are subtle, the condition can be overlooked.

Diabetes

If diabetes runs in your family, or you're middle-aged and you've been struggling with a weight problem for years, be sure your doctor tests your blood glucose levels to check for this disease. Weight problems can put you at risk for type 2 (also called *adult onset*) diabetes, which in turn can add pounds—in addition to putting you at risk for life-threatening complications.

While weight *loss* is often a first sign of type 1 diabetes, that's not necessarily true for type 2 diabetes. In fact, most people with this form of diabetes go undiagnosed for years because they have no early symptoms at all. This includes increasing numbers of children (see Step Ten), so it's important to ask your pediatrician to check for diabetes if your child is overweight.

The new diabetes drug metformin is helping many overweight people with diabetes take off excess pounds. (Interestingly, metformin also helps women with polycystic ovary syndrome. This is one exception to the "no diet drugs" rule, because metformin actually treats real medical problems—and weight loss is just a happy side effect!)

Other Conditions That Can Cause Weight Gain

Hormonal problems are among the most common medical causes of weight gain, but other conditions can cause you to put on pounds or have difficulty losing them. Among them are the following.

Taking Medications

Drugs are a double-edged sword: they can save your life or improve your quality of life, but they can also cause side effects. Several common prescription drugs, such as steroids and some psychotropic medications (used to treat psychiatric conditions), can cause substantial weight gain. Depo-Prevera, a form of birth control, also can cause many women to put on pounds. In addition, birth control pills and Depo-Prevera have been reported to cause depression, which can lead to overeating and weight gain.

Talk to your doctor if you are taking any medication, to find out (a) if the drug could be causing you to gain weight, (b) if there are acceptable substitutes, or (c) if the drug can safely be discontinued. Also, set realistic weight goals that take your medication's effects into account.

Sleep Apnea

If you have sleep apnea, you actually stop breathing for moments at a time. That's because your airway is narrow or obstructed and air can't flow easily in or out. During the day you're too exhausted to exercise and likely to overindulge in coffee, alcohol, or food as a means of keeping yourself awake or to combat anxiety. It's a vicious cycle in which apnea contributes to overeating and more weight gain, which in turn makes the apnea worse.

As many as twelve million Americans suffer from sleep apnea, and, again, most don't know that they have this serious problem. Problems associated with sleep apnea include:

overweight
snoring
chronic fatigue, depression, or irritability

Sleep apnea is usually easy to treat, with a simple breathing machine that helps force air into the lungs at night. If you have sleep apnea, you're likely to lose weight when you're treated, because you'll be healthier, happier, and more energetic.

Depression or Anxiety

Do you feel as if there's a dense fog separating you from the world you once enjoyed? Do you find the simplest tasks—picking out an outfit for work, making breakfast, walking the dog—hard to contemplate and often feel as though life is joyless? Or are you coping with extreme anxiety that makes your heart race and your hands tremble, keeps you awake at night, and frequently makes everyday life a nightmare?

Help Starts with Recognition

Are you suffering from depression, anxiety, or panic disorder? The first step in overcoming any of these disorders is to become aware of your symptoms and the impact they have on your life. While it's beyond the scope of this book to discuss these conditions at length, the following lists will help you spot possible signs and symptoms.

Signs and Symptoms of Depression

- Have you suffered, for more than two weeks, from depressed mood or loss of interest or pleasure?
- Do you experience a depressed mood most of the day, nearly every day?
- Have you lost interest or pleasure in life activities?
- Are you experiencing significant weight gain (or loss)?
- Do you oversleep or have trouble sleeping?
- Do you lack energy and feel tired nearly every day?
- Do you frequently experience feelings of worthlessness, guilt, or hopelessness?
- Are you finding it difficult to concentrate, think, or make decisions?
- Do you have recurrent thoughts of death or suicide?

Signs and Symptoms of Anxiety Disorder

- Do you suffer from excessive worry and anxiety on most days?
- Do you find it difficult or impossible to deal with your worries?
- Do you feel restless, "keyed up," or edgy?
- Do you feel stressed, tense, or fatigued?
- Do you have difficulty concentrating or find your mind going blank?
- Are you irritable?
- Do you have difficulty sleeping?

Signs and Symptoms of Panic Disorder

- Do you experience sudden, almost paralyzing attacks of panic?
- Do these attacks occur fairly regularly?
- During these attacks, do you feel that you may be losing your mind or that you are dying?
- When these attacks occur, do you experience a racing heartbeat, difficulty breathing, dizziness or light-headedness, and/or the feeling that you "can't get enough air"? Do you experience trembling, sweating, shaking, chest pains, hot flashes or chills, a "pins and needles" feeling in your fingers or toes, a choking sensation, and/or nausea?

Depression affects more than eighteen million Americans, and its crippling symptoms can interfere with your relationships, family life, and career or can even endanger your life. Anxiety disorders and panic disorder can be equally devastating, preventing you from leading a normal life and trapping you in your fears. These disorders often go hand-in-hand with weight problems, because food comforts and consoles us, and it's natural for us to eat when we're sad or frightened.

If you believe that you may be suffering from depression, anxiety, panic disorder, or any other psychiatric condition, it's crucial to seek professional help. Doctors now have powerful psychotherapeutic and medical treatments that can help free you from the devastating symptoms of these disorders.

One form of depression strongly linked to weight gain is seasonal affective disorder (SAD), stemming from lack of sunlight. As many as 8 percent of people in northern states suffer from SAD symptoms during the winter months.

If you have SAD, you may be sad and fatigued during dark days, and you're likely to crave carbohydrate foods, be irritable, and lose interest in sex. Many SAD sufferers put on ten, twenty, or even thirty pounds over the winter months and then gradually lose the weight in the spring and summer. (Gaining a few pounds in the winter is normal, no doubt a genetic legacy from our

Are You Suffering from SAD?

Many people who suffer from seasonal affective disorder experience the symptoms listed here. Answer the following questions and seek professional help if you believe that SAD may be a cause of your weight problems.

- Do you feel happy and have energy during the spring and summer but begin feeling fatigued and sad during the fall and winter, when the days are shorter?
- Do you crave high-carbohydrate foods such as pasta and bread during days of short sunlight?
- Is overeating a more severe problem for you in the winter than in the summer?
- Do you lose interest in sex during winter months?
- Do you have difficulty thinking and concentrating during the winter but not during the summer?
- Do you sleep more, or have more difficulty waking up, during the winter?

early ancestors, who needed extra padding to survive cold months. If you gain a great deal of weight each winter, however, SAD could be to blame.)

SAD is a highly treatable cause of depression and weight gain, so tell your doctor if you experience the symptoms listed in the "Are You Suffering from SAD?" sidebar. Your doctor may prescribe the natural remedy of increasing your exposure to light, either by getting more sun or by using a specially designed light box.

If you experience depression, anxiety, or other emotional or mental symptoms that make it hard for you to get through daily life, take control of your life by seeking help. The biggest tragedy of treatable mental disorders is that people suffer unnecessarily for years because they're embarrassed or ashamed to talk to their doctors. But secrecy about mental illness is as corrosive as secrecy about food and weight preoccupations (see Step Eight), and facing your problems openly and courageously is the first step toward freeing yourself. In addition, when you get effective treatment for depression or anxiety, you'll remove a major barrier to permanent fitness and weight loss.

Note: The symptoms I've described in this section can be signs of other medical conditions as well. If you are experiencing these symptoms or symptoms of any other psychiatric condition, it's crucial to obtain a complete evaluation immediately. It is always better to err on the side of safety, and your concerns may be beyond the scope of this book.

Take the Step

Your action plan in this step is simple: make the call! Pick up the phone, schedule an appointment, get a good checkup from a doctor you trust, and make sure that hidden health problems don't sabotage your reach for health and fitness.

And again, when you're in the doctor's office, be assertive and don't allow your physician to talk you into yet another thousand-calorie-a-day diet. *Note: If you have a medical condition that requires dietary limitations—for instance, diabetes or high blood pressure—be sure you understand these restrictions and follow them.* Also, refuse to accept any diet drugs unless it's clear that the advantages outweigh the risks—for instance, if you suffer from any medical condition that makes being overweight dangerous.

This is a good time, too, to talk with your doctor about any medical problems, such as knee or back problems, that could interfere with your exercise goals. Some of these problems are easy to correct, and if yours isn't, your doctor may be able to refer you to a physical therapist who can work with you to design a safe and fun fitness program.

When you get your checkup, you're likely to be reassured that you don't have any medical conditions that will make it hard for you to lose weight. But even if your doctor does uncover a medical problem, you'll be able to get effective treatment—and when you do, you'll have one less roadblock on your path to weight loss and a fit life.

Step Seven: Learn to Wait to Lose Weight

"Lose a dress size by next week!"
"Get the pill that melts off fat—take off twenty pounds in a single month."
"Be sixty pounds lighter by Christmas!"

YOU HEAR THESE claims every day—but the only way to attain a fit, sexy body for the rest of your life is to stop falling for them. In reality, to achieve a healthy and attractive weight you need to make a firm commitment to *accept gradual change*.

I know just how hard it is to accept this truth. Like you, I wanted to achieve the perfect body instantly. I took the diet pills, drank the shakes, ate the diet meals, and followed the killer exercise regimens, hoping that magically, miraculously, I could wake up six weeks later with a movie star's body. But it didn't work, and if you're reading this book, you probably already realize that it won't work for you.

What will work? *Losing weight healthily and permanently by losing it gradually.* It won't take forever to lose extra pounds, but it will take months—or, if you want to lose a very large amount of weight, possibly even longer—to achieve your body's ideal weight. But this time, when you lose the weight, it will stay off for good.

Why Fast Weight Loss Leads to Failure

If you've tried "quick weight loss" diets, you know the truth: when you lose pounds quickly, you put them back on just as fast. Worse yet, when you end a diet, you usually gain back more weight than you lost. That's because your body reacts to an intense period of semistarvation by making you crave large amounts of "forbidden" high-calorie, high-fat, high-carbohydrate foods. (For a more in-depth explanation, see Chapter 2.)

Thousands of years of evolution have taught your body that starvation is dangerous. Because of this, you react to a restricted diet in the same way as your Neanderthal ancestors did: you grow ravenously hungry, because your body wants you to store extra fat. Worse, your body goes into survival mode, slowing your metabolism, hoarding fat, and even putting on water weight to make weight loss harder. Your body doesn't know that your food shortage is artificial; it thinks there's a real danger that you'll starve to death, and it pulls out all the stops in an effort to save you.

Even when you "wise up" and stop dieting, it takes time to reset your metabolism so you can burn calories more easily. Chronic dieting sends your body the message "Conserve body fat at all costs!" To reverse this process, you need to convince your body that the danger of starvation is over—and that won't happen overnight.

In addition, you need to allow time for both your body and your mind to recover from the stress of dieting. New research shows that stress itself can put on pounds, which is another reason the ordeal of dieting usually results, ironically, in added weight and inches. To understand this pattern, let's look at how stress changes your body in ways that promote weight gain—and why it takes time to reverse this process.

The Stress-Weight Cycle

You start a new diet, feeling powerful and optimistic. You believe in your heart that this diet will be different. It's guaranteed to speed your metabolism, alter your body chemistry, burn the pounds off.

You follow the diet religiously for weeks. You brag to your friends about how much weight you're losing. Your mother says, encouragingly, "I can't wait to take you shopping when you lose another size!" You think, This time I'm going to make it. You feel strong and in control.

Then, inevitably, it happens. Your weight loss slows and then stops. Worse, you begin to crave the "bad" foods your diet forbids, and you feel empty and unsatisfied when you eat the "good" foods it allows. You expend more and more energy fighting your growing urges to eat. Increasingly, you feel anxious, tired, even hopeless.

Eventually, you go off the diet for a day . . . then two days. Each day you find it harder and harder to avoid ice cream or chocolate or spaghetti. Your weight creeps up. You're ashamed to see your friends, because you know they'll notice. Your mother says, "Don't worry, dear. We all know you tried." Within a few weeks you gain back all the weight you lost, and five pounds more—and the stress of dieting is replaced by the stress of wondering, "Will I keep gaining weight no matter what I do?"

Dieting is traumatic. It puts enormous stress on your body, triggering survival mechanisms that drastically alter its chemistry. In addition, it puts enormous stress on you psychologically. Each time you begin a diet, you invest your energy, pride, and self-esteem in the effort, and each failure takes a psychic toll.

Research shows, too, that the stress-linked effects of dieting don't end when you stop. That's because when you expose your mind and body to chronic stress, as you do when you diet repetitively and endure the emotional pain of each failure, your body produces excess levels of the "stress hormone" cortisol—and changes in cortisol levels can cause long-term alterations in your appetite and metabolism.

Research shows that cortisol levels rise not just in extreme dieters and bingers but in typical dieters, too. A recent study of sixty-two women showed that "high food restrictors" exhibited significantly higher cortisol levels than "low food restrictors," a finding the researchers hypothesize is due to "the psychological stress of constantly trying to monitor and control food intake."[1]

Studies link elevated cortisol levels, in turn, to increased appetite and weight gain. For example:

- In one experiment, scientists asked women to perform stressful tasks (for instance, solving an impossible puzzle or giving a speech) and measured their saliva cortisol levels. Afterward, they provided a choice of high-fat and low-fat snacks to the women. The women who secreted the most cortisol ate the highest-fat foods after the stressful experience, while those who secreted the least cortisol selected lower-fat snacks.[2]

- Scientists studying "night bingeing," in which people awaken during the night and eat, found that night bingers have unusually high night-time cortisol levels.[3]
- Another study found that participants in a weight-loss program reported increased appetites and that "the most consistent predictor of these changes in appetite seems to be changes in fasting plasma cortisol."[4]
- Increased cortisol is seen in Cushing's syndrome and sometimes in polycystic ovary syndrome, conditions associated with increased weight (see Step Six).

When your cortisol levels are high because of the stress of dieting, it takes time for them to drop to normal levels. It's important to recognize this when you stop dieting so you don't add to your stress by expecting instant results. You don't want to fight your body chemistry; you want it to work with you!

So allow time for your body to recognize that it's no longer stressed or starving and to adjust your metabolism and lower your cortisol levels in response. When this happens, the excess pounds will eventually begin to come off easily and naturally.

Putting It in Perspective

Here's a good way to look at dieting versus my no-diet fitness plan. If you continue to diet, the number of months you spend on diets that *don't work* will add up to years over time—and statistics say, consistently and with nearly 100 percent certainty, that you'll wind up weighing just as much or more over the long run. *It takes far less time to lose the weight successfully, by losing it gradually, than it does to yo-yo for years and never reach your goal!*

If you're skeptical, I'm not surprised. We're all indoctrinated by the diet industry to believe in "miracle diets" that take off pounds instantly. But you know, from your own experience, that miracle diets don't work. To lose weight permanently, you need to accept a radically different idea: that you can lose weight naturally and permanently, without fads or gimmicks, if you're willing to be patient.

Losing Weight in a Stressful World

Dieting isn't good for your body *or* your weight, and as you eliminate the stress of diet regimens, the pounds will gradually start to come off more and more effortlessly. But dieting isn't the only stress trigger in your life. We all cope with job pressures, money worries, family tensions, illnesses, and other stressors that can make us eat when we're not hungry.

You'll need to have patience while your body heals from the stress of dieting, but you can facilitate this healing by recognizing the additional stressors that affect you and taking positive steps to deal with them before they can sabotage your fitness plan.

During my second pregnancy I gained thirty pounds. I thought losing the weight would be simple; after all, I'd gained a modest amount for a full-term pregnancy.

I returned to work eight weeks after my daughter was born, tackling a demanding, high-stress job at a busy public psychiatric hospital. I worked late almost every day, never had time for lunch, woke up tense and anxious, and fell into bed exhausted each night. Then I accepted an even more demanding job that took even more of my time and energy. During this time I couldn't understand why the pounds I'd gained during pregnancy didn't melt away. After all, since I had stopped dieting and learned to eat naturally, I'd had no trouble controlling my weight.

I discovered the answer when I decided to leave my high-pressure job and work part-time. During the summer that followed my job change, the extra seven or eight pounds melted off my body without effort. No doubt the summer sunlight helped (see my discussion about seasonal affective disorder in Chapter 9), but I'm sure that reducing my stress level helped even more.

In a world that's full of pressure and tension, how can you avoid being stressed? You can't, but you can change how you deal with stress. Mild or moderate exercise reduces tension and produces "feel good" chemicals called *endorphins* that can counter the effects of stress. Taking time for yourself— for a hot bath, a movie, or an hour of reading—allows your mind and body to unwind.

In addition, consider simplifying your life, especially if you're trying to juggle a career and family. Reevaluate your job, your volunteer commitments, your financial obligations, and even your holiday expectations and see if you can cut out stressful activities that aren't worth the effort and anxiety. (Do you *really* want to be PTA president? Will your friends care if you send E-cards, or skip holiday card mailing altogether, instead of laboring over handwritten cards?)

If you find that you're tense all the time, you'll find more good suggestions for "destressing" your life in a wonderful book by Elaine St. James called *Simplify Your Life: 100 Ways to Slow Down and Enjoy the Things That Really Matter.* If your stress is serious and chronic, you may need to reevaluate your career and your relationships and make some significant changes—as I did, when I changed my lifestyle to focus on my own needs and my family's.

Be Patient with Yourself During Stressful Times

As you make the commitment to accept gradual weight loss, make a commitment to be patient and loving with yourself as well. That means being accepting of yourself if you temporarily stop losing weight, or even gain a few pounds, during stressful periods. I talked earlier about the crucial role that self-acceptance plays in permanent weight loss, but I cannot overstate the importance of accepting and loving yourself during difficult periods in your life. Now, while your body is going through physiological and emotional changes, is the time to remain committed to the act of being patient and kind to yourself.

If you are grieving over the death of someone you love or dealing with a job loss, an illness, the breakup of a relationship, or another stressful life change, you may be more at risk for emotional eating. It will require mental concentration and self-awareness to recognize that this is not a sign of failure but a natural human response to pain or distress and to avoid stressful self-criticism and negative thoughts if this occurs.

You may find it hard to remain positive when stress or suffering saps your energy, morale, and self-esteem. Realize, however, that this fitness program

What You Can Do While You Wait:
Tips for Mindful Eating

Remember that losing weight and becoming fit require work, defined as "mental and physical energy directed toward a goal." This is an active—not passive—process, and it requires you to concentrate on yourself and on your needs. The good news? Unlike the demoralizing work involved in dieting, this work will be directed toward consciously noticing and respecting your needs, rather than ignoring them (which, for most of us, leads to a state of physical and emotional deprivation, and ultimately, to weight gain). Losing weight also requires making your own fitness and well-being a *priority* in your life.

Here are some practical day-to-day suggestions that will help you stay focused and avoid falling back into old traps of dieting or unconsciously overeating.

- Each day, take a shower (even if you're staying home), and dress in clothes that you enjoy wearing. Be sure to have plenty of clothes that you like in your size. It's crucial to learn to respect and care for your body, no matter what size you are.
- If possible, brush your teeth following each meal, after you feel satiated. If you have a tendency to "zone out" after you eat, this helps you "wake up" and maintain the awareness that you're full. If you realize that you are not satiated, or you become hungry again, it's fine to eat even if you've already brushed your teeth.
- Don't mistake thirst for hunger. If you're very thirsty, be sure to drink water rather than something that artificially satisfies your thirst sensation, such as coffee or carbonated drinks.
- Limit or avoid alcohol, and stay drug-free. Alcohol and drug use tend to cause us to be less focused and aware of our inner state and ourselves and can have damaging physical and psychological effects. Ask for help if you need it. (continued)

- At least twice a week, engage in some form of relaxing activity that integrates your mind and body—for example, a facial, a massage, yoga, stretching, meditation, a Jacuzzi, or a steam/sauna. Be sure it's an activity that you actually enjoy and can look forward to.
- If you're medically able to do so, start walking on a regular basis.
- Engage each morning in a moment of quiet, making a vow during this time to *remain conscious of your inner state* all day.
- If you like jewelry, accessories, or perfume, occasionally buy something nice for yourself.
- Do each day what you would do if you were at the size and weight that you feel is ideal for you.
- Be as kind, gentle, and respectful of yourself as you would be to another who has walked in your path.
- Periodically reread the steps that you find the most challenging. This may be especially helpful during stressful times such as holidays, job changes, moves, and relationship break-ups, or during times of hormonal changes.

is different from dieting, because your goal is to focus on the self-awareness and self-fulfillment that are the real keys to achieving long-term weight loss. (I've often thought that if people spent half as much energy on identifying and addressing their inner state as they spend on counting calories and dieting, we could virtually eliminate America's epidemic of excess weight.)

Part of the process of change involves *facing obstacles and enduring setbacks*, and only when you can persevere and continue in spite of these challenges can you succeed. You are on the path to true fitness and health, and if the path takes a few twists and turns, you *will* still reach your goal!

Realize, too, that aging, medical conditions, medication use (see Step Six), and other factors can affect how fast your body is able to shed extra pounds. If you're a woman, recognize that it's harder to lose weight after a pregnancy or during menopause. If you're a man, understand that weight loss takes more time as you reach middle age. In addition, your genes have an important say in how easily your body loses or gains weight and what your realistic ideal weight will be. The pounds will come off, but they will come off on your body's schedule—so be patient.

Wait to Change, Not to Live

When I look back on the days when I dieted, some memories sadden me. I realize that for more than a decade I put my life on hold, refusing to give myself permission to live life fully and joyously until the magical day when a miracle diet would make my hated pounds disappear. Like the fictitious heroine in *Bridget Jones's Diary*, I believed if I could simply transform my "flabby, flobbering around" body (to borrow Bridget's words) into a model-like shape, I could become a new woman—somehow more worthy, happier, more fulfilled. Even as each diet failed, I eagerly bought into the claims of the next one, believing that my salvation lay in becoming a different, thinner person. Similarly, many repetitive dieters fool themselves into believing that the newest quick-fix diet, whatever it is, will be the one that finally transforms them into a new person—one capable of being loved and happy and one who can really enjoy and live life.

As a result of this diet mentality, we throw away precious and irreplaceable time. When I recall my years of dieting and bingeing, my memories don't include many unadulterated joys, pleasures, and new experiences. Instead I see a parade of memories about weight . . . about dieting . . . about being hungry . . . about bingeing alone and suffering in secrecy.

If you find yourself trapped by the idea that your life won't start until you lose weight, don't make the mistake I made. Instead make a decision, right now, to *own your life in the present.* Don't sacrifice another precious day of your life to the numbers on your bathroom scale. Don't throw away today, believing that you cannot be happy until you look like a model or movie star. Doing so won't help (and will probably harm) your efforts to lose weight, and the physical and emotional costs will be enormous.

Instead, consider it possible that beauty comes in many forms and that you can choose not to be trapped by a socially driven, unnaturally narrow definition of attractiveness. Moreover, you can live your life to the fullest even *while* you make positive changes in your weight, appearance, and fitness.

Say Good-Bye to Your Scale

When you throw out the idea that you "must" lose a specific amount of weight by a specific date, consider discarding another symbol of your old diet mentality along with it: your bathroom scale. At the very least, put your scale in the closet and avoid weighing yourself more than once or twice a month.

Your body weight normally fluctuates from day to day and even from week to week, so short-term weight changes are virtually meaningless. And if you're trimming off fat pounds and gaining lean muscle, the numbers on your scale may actually go up at times, even while you're losing inches. Thus constant scale hopping tells you nothing about your real weight loss, and it can cause a tremendous amount of unnecessary stress and anxiety. You can gain a better idea of your progress by noticing the fit of your clothes or the changes you see in the mirror.

Also avoid trying to "speed up" your weight loss by turning this fitness plan into yet another stressful diet—for instance, by restricting certain foods or by saying to yourself, "I'll lose ten pounds each month on the **Fed Up** plan." Relax: the pounds will come off, and they'll come off more easily if you make a clean break from old dieting habits.

When you fully realize these powerful truths, you will be surprised at how much easier weight loss becomes.

I am reminded, as I write this, of a remark that one of my wonderful colleagues, psychologist Barbara Kohlenberg, made recently. Mentioning that she'd been invited to give a talk on self-improvement, she told me that she planned to talk about self-acceptance instead—because the key to self-improvement is self-acceptance and accepting the process of change.

As you realize this truth, and see that there is more to your life than what you weigh, you will gradually stop being obsessed about food and discover more important interests, goals, and pleasures that will allow you to accept gradual weight loss. As a result, *you will lose weight far more successfully than when you dieted*—and you will live each day to the fullest, while taking pleasure in your changing body. In addition, by freeing yourself from the stress-producing and unrealistic idea that your happiness depends on instant weight loss, you will begin to break the biological cycle of stress and weight gain.

As psychologist Erich Fromm noted, "Modern man thinks he loses something—time—when he does not do things quickly; yet he does not know what to do with the time he gains—except kill it."[5] Resolve not to kill time by living a half-life until the imaginary day when you will become model thin. Instead, make a firm commitment to be patient with yourself and your body as you gradually lose weight and to enjoy every day to the fullest—both before and after you achieve the body you desire.

Part IV

Steps Eight Through Ten

Reach Out and Share Your Strength

IN STEPS EIGHT through Ten I challenge you to connect with other important people in your life and in the world around you in a new, healthier way. You'll discover to your surprise that this generative action will help you keep weight off permanently as it strengthens you and brings new joy and meaning to your life.

Step Eight: Break Through the Secrecy

"I would literally empty a refrigerator. I spent most of every day either thinking about food, shopping for food, or bingeing and purging."

Actress Jane Fonda, who concealed her eating problems from
friends and the public for more than two decades[1]

It was a Friday night, and I sat in my dorm room, alone. I'd eaten only a few hundred calories since morning, barely enough to keep my body functioning through a long day of classes.

All around me, students laughed and yelled, ran down hallways, whispered excitedly about Friday-night plans, worried about grades, complained about the overcooked cafeteria food, primped for dates. Behind my closed door there was silence, except for my worried thoughts. How much had I eaten that day? Had I lost any weight? Could I make it through the weekend without bingeing?

It was my sophomore year at college, and I was lonely, but slowly making friends. Recently I'd met a nice guy named Greg who drove a fancy sports car and loved to play backgammon. On this night, however, I wasn't thinking about Greg. Food was the only thing on my mind.

I was desperately hungry. In fact, in retrospect, I can see that I was actually physically starving, but I'd dieted for too many years to know how to respond normally to this sensation. Instead, feeling lonely and anxious, I went for a walk. Not surprisingly, I wound up at the nearest grocery store. From there, as if on psychic autopilot, I went to an ice cream store and then a McDonald's, returning to my dorm room with bags of candy, ice cream, and fast food. As I locked my door, a comforting thought, the necessary precursor to each binge, loomed beneath the surface of my mind: Nobody is watching. Sitting on my floor, I began an eating frenzy. It doesn't matter, I told myself. I'll go running tomorrow. I'll be good tomorrow.

Euphoria exploded within me as I broke through the steel barrier in my mind that prohibited me from eating. A rush flowed through my soul as I detached from the world, gobbling down the food until my stomach was swollen and I felt sick.

FOR PEOPLE WITH FOOD and body preoccupations, secrecy is a way of life. We eat salads in public and then furtively gobble ice cream or leftover mashed potatoes in the middle of the night. We hide in bathrooms, frantically stuffing ourselves with "forbidden" candy bars. Some of us sneak off to purge ourselves after a big meal.

We are secretive, because we believe we have something to hide—something shameful. We are ashamed of our desire to eat and our loss of control when we eat. If we binge, we do so in hiding, like hunted animals. If we become anorexic, we hide the fact that we *don't* eat. Even those of us who say we've given up on weight control and "don't care anymore" what others think of us tend to eat behind closed doors, when no one is watching.

No matter what pattern our eating or dieting takes, our shame creates a divide between the world and ourselves. We raid the refrigerator at night, when everyone else is sleeping, so no one will see us breaking our diets. We sneak into markets to buy "forbidden" cookies or chips, feeling as guilty as shoplifters. Those of us with eating disorders hide in bathrooms to purge ourselves or put food down the disposal when no one is looking. Already ashamed of our bodies, we compound our lack of self-acceptance with the guilt we feel when we deceive our friends and families in a desperate attempt to cover up our behavior.

"It's the shame and the secrecy . . . that cut the deepest," one bulimic confided in her school newspaper. "Running water and cranking the music to muffle the gagging and choking. . . . Making excuses about why I seem to be losing weight, why I spend so much time in the bathroom, and why the groceries disappear so quickly." Similarly, the overweight woman who hides in the basement to eat half a chocolate pie, the teenage dieter who sneaks her mother's home-cooked meal into the trash, and the young male bodybuilder who breaks his regimen to secretly scarf down a pizza feel degraded, both by their behavior and by the lies they tell about it.

> *I awoke from my binge—I think of it as awakening because the sensation of coming back to reality was so similar to the sensation of awakening from a dream. I felt low and horrible, as I had so many times before. Then the self-blame began: How could I have done it? What a pig I was! I looked at myself in the mirror and felt disgust. I was overwhelmed by guilt and shame.*
>
> *Just then I heard a knock on my door. It was Greg, asking if I wanted to play backgammon.*
>
> *I panicked. There were greasy hamburger wrappers all over my room. An empty container of praline ice cream lay on the bed. The spoon I'd used to eat the ice cream lay on the floor, where I'd sat wolfing food insatiably. Candy wrappers were strewn about.*
>
> *Quickly, I shoved everything under my bed, wondering if my room smelled in the aftermath of my binge. I wanted to hide in my room, but I knew Greg had heard me inside, so I opened the door.*
>
> *I felt hideous, and all I could think of was to get rid of this nice young man who wanted to have fun with me. I told him I had schoolwork due on Monday and had to study. He was disappointed, and I sensed that he didn't believe me. He offered to take me for a ride in his car . . . for ice cream! If only he knew what was under my bed.*

When I hid the evidence of my binge from Greg, I did so because I saw the grease-stained wrappers and ice cream–covered napkins as signs that I was disgusting or even unbalanced. Similarly, you may hide candy bars in your clothes hamper or binge in the privacy of your car, because you feel ashamed about your behavior or even fearful that you are "acting crazy." Even if you don't binge, but merely "sneak" a piece of pie or a biscuit now and then, you may do so guiltily and secretively, when no one is looking.

The shame and secrecy that are almost universal among dieters, bingers, and overeaters is a logical, perhaps even inevitable, result of the distorted role that food plays in our lives. This is particularly true for women, who are taught from our earliest days that feminine women don't eat "too much." This prohibition is a powerful one, and few women dare to disobey it. If we are dating, we order tiny meals, carefully time our bites so that we stretch out our meals, and say, "Oh, I'm so full" even if we're still hungering for more. If we are caregivers, we nurture our husbands and families with beautifully prepared meals while grabbing "just a bite" between serving and cleaning the table. We spend hours in the kitchen each day, preparing food that we forbid ourselves to touch. As eating disorders expert Susan Bordo notes, we are bound by the cultural stricture "Men eat and women prepare." Our appetites, she says, are artificially restricted by "the notion that women are most gratified by feeding and nourishing others, not themselves."

The media continually reinforce the idea that hearty eating is acceptable or even desirable for men but taboo for women. Commercials show men heartily devouring fried chicken or apple pie, while women rhapsodize over the thrill of eating tiny low-calorie cookies. Ads invite men to savor the experience of eating half-pound steaks or honey-drenched biscuits, while portraying women as angelic for restricting themselves to tiny squares of cheesecake. And again and again, we see women serving meals to men and children while almost never eating—or even sitting down at the table—themselves.

The messages are all too clear: Food is fun for men, dangerous for women. Women gain pleasure from serving food, not from eating it. And when women do eat, the only acceptable foods are tiny in size or low in calories.

Conditioned by these messages, we buy in to the concept that semistarvation and femininity are inextricably linked. On dates we eat salads (no avocado, dressing on the side) while the men sitting across from us feast on lobster and steak. At the movie we ask for a mineral water and low-calorie jujubes instead of enjoying buttered popcorn or Junior Mints. We feed our families roasts and burgers and pizza and then drink diet milk shakes as we clear the table. The result: by the end of the day, we feel physical hunger we cannot assuage and emotional hunger we cannot heal.

And so we binge. But we binge in private, hiding what we perceive as grotesque and unwomanly gluttony. We sneak into the kitchen at midnight and wolf leftovers from plastic containers. We hide in the bathroom, running the bathwater so no one will hear us. We eat in dorm rooms with our doors locked. We hide in cars, in the dark, parked behind fast-food restaurants, ducking our heads so passersby will not see us. We drive to different neighborhoods so people who know that we're dieting won't see us "blow it."

And even if we don't binge, we feel shame each time we abandon a diet, trading in our carrot sticks and rice cakes for the foods we crave. We wonder what our friends and family will think if they see us eating hamburgers or pizza or if they notice that we've gained back the pounds we worked so hard to lose. So we admit defeat, but we hide our shame and embarrassment by indulging in macaroni and cheese, ice cream, or hash browns only when we're safely alone, with no one to judge us but ourselves. Just as I hid alone in my dorm room to binge, we hide ourselves away to eat—and our secrecy feeds our sickness, exacerbating the disease of dieting.

Secrecy and the Male with Food and Body Preoccupations

For men, unlike women, food and eating are not ingrained cultural taboos. To the majority of men a piece of cake is merely a piece of cake—fattening, perhaps, but not an object with the power to define them as good or bad. Moreover, our culture is more realistic about the "ideal" male body than the "ideal" female body. As a result, far fewer men than women develop eating disorders. Yet in an age when appearance is all-important, increasing numbers of males—athletes in sports where weight is critical, gay men, bodybuilders, actors, dancers, middle-aged men afraid of aging, young men who've battled weight problems since childhood—are falling prey to the same food preoccupations that drive women to diet repetitively.

For the men who do develop food preoccupations, the stigma is enormous, largely because anorexia, bulimia, and overeating are labeled as "girl problems." The director of Support, Concern, and Resources for Eating Disorders (SCaRED), a support group for people with eating disorders, tells of a person who contacted her using the name Tracy but later confessed that he was male. "His fear of being rejected or snickered at by others left him to suffer

Building Bulimics: A Laboratory Experiment

Dieting continually reinforces our negative self-images—"I'm weak," "I'm crazy," "I'm disgusting." We diet in secret and eat in secret because we believe that "normal" people would never act as we do: hoarding and hiding food, obsessing constantly about food and eating, alternating between starving ourselves and wolfing down food when our control breaks down.

But here is a surprise: that's *exactly* what people who have healthy eating habits and no weight issues begin doing when they're put on diets, according to scientists! The remarkable proof comes from a classic study, reported back in the 1950s.

Ancel Keys and his colleagues asked thirty-six young men, chosen for their superb mental and physical health, to live for six months on half of their normal food intake. (Their calorie intake, while defined as "semistarvation," is typical for an American dieter.) After the diet phase the researchers studied how the men adjusted to normal eating again.

What happened to these perfectly healthy, bright, psychologically well-adjusted men over the course of the experiment?

- **They became obsessed with thoughts of food and eating.** "Those who ate in the common dining room," Keys reported, "smuggled out bits of food and consumed them on their bunks in a long, drawn-out ritual."
- **They binged.** During the dieting phase they sneaked or even stole food. During the "refeeding" phase they "ate more or less continuously," frequently to the point of illness. (In fact one required hospitalization after a severe binge.)
- **They experienced self-disgust.** Keys described one man, for instance, who "suffered a complete loss of will power and ate several cookies, a sack of popcorn, and two overripe bananas

before he could 'regain control' of himself. He immediately suffered a severe emotional upset, with nausea, and upon returning
to the laboratory he vomited. . . . He was self-deprecatory,
expressing disgust and self-criticism."

In short, *the dieting patterns we see in ourselves—hoarding food,
bingeing, self-disgust—can actually be created in the laboratory, simply
by putting normal (or, in this case, even healthier than normal) people on
a severely restricted diet.*

Why is this so crucial to understand? Because it means there is no
reason to be ashamed of your behavior. You are not abnormal. You
are not disgusting. You are not weak. You are not weird or crazy.
Instead you are a perfectly normal individual, with a dangerous but
curable problem: the culturally inflicted disease called *dieting.* Your
behavior, while it seems disgusting or even frightening, is an understandable and expected reaction to the effects of dieting. It is your
mind's and body's way of fighting to return to a normal life.

in secrecy and loneliness," she says. "It is almost like he has been victimized
once by his eating disorder, and secondly by society."

Additionally, many heterosexual men with eating disorders or food and
body problems hide their condition for fear that friends will believe that they
are gay or unmasculine if they are worried about their bodies. (Interestingly,
gay men, while they suffer from eating disorders in higher numbers than
straight men, sometimes find it easier to open up about their problem and to
seek help—perhaps because members of the gay community are more accustomed to confronting and overcoming social stigma.)

One result of men's extreme secrecy about food obsessions is that the incidence of eating disorders in males may be grossly underestimated. A recent survey found that the prevalence of eating disorders among navy personnel
assigned to hospitals and clinics was 2.5 percent for anorexia and 6.8 percent
for bulimia. Twenty-seven percent of the men who responded to the survey
reported that they had engaged in binge eating over the past three months.[2]

The remarkably high incidence of disordered eating in this group of men, who do not belong to groups considered to be at risk for food obsession, is a strong indication that many thousands of men in the general population may be "hidden" sufferers who conceal their disordered eating.

Overcoming Our Destructive Shame

Years ago, as a resident at Bellevue Hospital in New York City, I worked every fourth night in the psychiatric emergency room. While many of the patients brought to us were severely mentally ill, patients from certain cultures tended to be brought to the hospital in much worse condition than the other patients.

One night, when I was on call with an experienced psychiatrist, he offered an explanation for this. In some cultures, he told me, people with mental illness are stigmatized particularly harshly. In fact, if a family member is discovered to be mentally ill, it can affect the entire extended family, whose members may find it difficult to marry. Thus, the psychiatrist explained, the family of a person who becomes mentally ill often will do everything within their power to avoid exposing the problem to the community, keeping the affected individual hidden away.

The result, frequently, was that by the time these patients' symptoms grew so severe that their families could not hide the truth, the disease had progressed to the point where the patients were severely disoriented, psychotic, and very difficult to treat.

It struck me, as I thought about what he was saying, how similar my dieting behavior was to the behavior of these patients and their families. Their cultures taught them to hide their obsessions, their hallucinations, and their depression, while mine taught me to hide my eating, my bingeing, my purging, and my obsession with thinness. And, like them, the more I hid, the sicker I became.

Repetitive dieting is a disease that traps many of us in a web of food preoccupation and secrecy and leads others of us to give up on the idea of healthy weight loss and become furtive, guilt-ridden overeaters. But the secrets that we hide don't lie quietly. Instead they fester, damaging our self-esteem and distorting our relationships with others.

How do we cure the sickness of dieting or its counterpart, overeating? One of the first and most important steps is to open up to someone we love and trust. By hiding our food preoccupations, we magnify our problem and our guilt. When we take the brave step of sharing our secret with others, a remarkable thing happens: food and body preoccupations begin to lose their control over us.

I know, however, just how big a step I am asking you to take. I can clearly remember my own fears when I decided to tell my family members about my repetitive dieting and bingeing. They thought of me as the strong, successful one, and I was terrified of altering that image. Would they lose respect for me? Would I see my own self-image, that of a gluttonous pig with no self-control, reflected in their eyes?

Fortunately, none of my fears materialized. My brothers, whose concern and compassion I needed the most, were loving and accepting. I found that when I admitted my problem openly, my family respected me just as much as they had before, if not more. By releasing my burden of secrecy, I gained powerful allies in my battle against food preoccupation—and by ending the secrecy and the hiding and the lying, I regained my dignity as well.

As you open up to a trusted friend or relative, you will discover the remarkable power embodied in the simple act of transforming "shameful" secrets into shared feelings. However, while your goal in this step is to confide in a friend or family member, be careful not to cast that person in the role of therapist. Instead, simply acknowledge, with the people you trust and who are important to you, that you are facing a challenging, meaningful, and complex problem.

Of course, not every family member is capable of being supportive. Some of you are coping with abusive or dysfunctional families who are likely to respond negatively if you open up and talk honestly with them. If you believe that your family members cannot respond to your feelings in a loving and helpful way, talk instead with a trusted friend who is supportive and understanding. Or, if you do not feel ready to discuss your food and eating preoccupations with someone close to you, talk with a therapist or join a support group. (For other ideas, see the exercises at the end of this chapter.) It's crucial that the person you confide in be someone who will be understanding, positive, and likely to support your new approach—for instance, a close friend who's witnessed the toll that useless dieting has taken on your life.

An added benefit of confiding in a trusted friend is that this person often can help you identify eating patterns or triggers that you have difficulty spotting. A friend of mine, for instance, called me recently to express her concerns about her overeating. As we talked, she told me about her experiences living in a new country and about the stress of adjusting to new foods and new customs. Sorting through her feelings, she realized the triggers of her overeating episodes: stress, unfamiliar and often unsatisfying foods, and a need for comfort during a time of transition. Using me as a friendly sounding board, she identified both the problem and the solution—which was to spend more time getting in touch with her feelings and to plan her meals ahead so she'd be able to find food she enjoyed.

Advice for Friends and Family

Some of you are reading this book because you're a friend, partner, or relative of someone who's said, "I'm tired of dieting, bingeing, or overeating, and I'm trying this new plan. Please support me."

If so, you should be pleased that this person values and trusts you enough to share this important journey with you. But you're probably also wondering what you can do and say to help. If so, here's some advice:

• **Read all of the steps so you'll know what the person you're supporting is doing and why.** Become educated about the deleterious effects of dieting, and educate other family members as well, so that they will understand why the person who's undertaking this plan is saying "no" to diets. This is critical, because negative attitudes on the part of family members and friends can create anxiety and interfere with the person's healing and weight loss.

• **Understand the toll that weight and body issues are taking on the person's life.** Avoid trivializing the importance of the person's struggle with repetitive dieting or overeating.

• **Get rid of the toxic idea that the person you want to help is "guilty" of being overweight.** Weight problems do not stem from weakness or lack of willpower. (See Chapter 2 for more information.)

• **Be there and be positive.** Your friend, partner, or relative needs to overcome years of failed dieting and weight gain. Like any major positive life change, this will take time, work, and concentration. You can help by allowing the individual to share his or her feelings, successes, fears, and progress with you.

Unhelpful "Help"

Even the nicest people sometimes say counterproductive things when you talk with them about weight and food issues. It's important to set limits on this type of behavior, because it's hurtful and can interfere with your progress.

Here are some of the most common examples of "unhelpful helping" that my patients report and some of my favorite ways of countering them:

"Do you really think you can get thin eating *that*?"

- "Watch me!"
- "Well, I got overweight by *not* eating what I wanted . . . doesn't that tell you something?"

"Do you really need that ice cream?"

- "What I really need is for you to read this chapter on the medical effects of dieting and food restriction. When you're more knowledgeable about the current scientific findings, we'll talk."

"You'd be so beautiful if you lost some weight."

- "Hmmm, that's strange . . . my other friends think I'm beautiful now."

Sometimes, of course, the person who says something cruel or simply ignorant is a medical professional. Two of the worst lines my patients have heard from other doctors are "You're fat every day, so you should exercise every day" and "You've really let yourself go—would this happen if you were still single?" While you might be able to conjure up a snappy comeback to such ignorant comments, it's smarter simply to say "good-bye," and look for a new doctor who's wiser and more empathetic.

One reason that people coping with weight and body issues remain secretive is that they've been the targets of so many verbal slaps in the face. Your job is to offer verbal hugs and pats on the back instead—as well as your love, your respect, and your understanding.

Ending the Abusive Hold of Dieting and Body Preoccupation

There are times in life when we have good reason to feel ashamed or to keep secrets. The secrecy of people with food preoccupations, however, is misguided and self-destructive. We hide our behavior because we believe that we are at fault—but *we are not*.

In reality, our shame is similar to that of children victimized by sexual abuse. These children feel intense shame and frequently hide the fact that they are being abused. They feel that they must somehow be guilty of provoking the abuse—otherwise, why would it happen to them? And the more secretive they become, the longer the abuse and victimization continue.

Similarly, your out-of-control eating is not a behavior you freely choose but an almost unavoidable consequence of the abuse we call *dieting*. Blaming yourself for your food preoccupations is less logical than blaming the doctor who puts you on diets year after year; or the diet experts who push low-cal, low-carb, or fasting diets; or the diet-pill dispensers who relentlessly spread the message that their drugs and "a little willpower" can transform you into a model-thin goddess. You are not the guilty party in this scenario, but rather the abused party—and your starving, bingeing, overeating, shame, and secret guilt are the results of this abuse.

Moreover, just as an abused child's secrecy leads to more abuse, your silence increases the hold that dieting or overeating possesses over you. Secrecy and shame breed low self-esteem, leading you right back to the refrigerator and the next binge.

Conversely, each time you share your experiences with someone you can trust, you loosen the grip that food and body preoccupation holds over your life. Moreover, you may be amazed—as I was—by the number of friends and family members who say, "I'm so glad you told me. I have the same problem—and I need someone to talk to."

Say "Good-Bye" to Shame: Exercises in Reaching Out, Giving, and Receiving

The following exercises will help you find support and resources.

Surf the Net

Locate Internet groups where people coping with repetitive dieting, overeating, or eating disorders can share their experiences. (I recommend somethingfishy.org as a good starting point. See "Resources" for more.) It's OK simply to "lurk" and read what others are saying. Eventually, however, you may want to try posting messages about your own experiences. This is an excellent first step out of your secrecy, because you can remain anonymous while relating your experiences to an understanding group of individuals struggling with the same issues as you.

Journal

Begin a diary of your binges or episodes of overeating. Write down how you felt before, during, and after each episode. Do not be judgmental. Rather, be open with yourself about your feelings and experience—a first step toward being open toward others.

As you write in your diary, see if you detect clues about the pattern of your overeating or bingeing—for instance, do you reach for food to ease your anxiety before stressful events or major changes in your life? If you're female, do you tend to binge during the week before your period starts? As you realize that bingeing or overeating is your mind's way of seeking comfort or nurturing during difficult times, and not a sign that you are "weak" or "bad," you will feel less destructive guilt, shame, and secrecy.

Check Out Your Local Bookstore or Library

Read books by men or women who have suffered from binge eating, overeating, or eating disorders. (Among those I recommend is Kim Chernin's *The Hungry Self: Women, Eating, and Identity*. See "Resources" for more.) Observe how they are now able to discuss, openly and without shame, the feelings and behaviors that they once concealed from others.

Share Your Struggle

When you believe that you are ready, sit down with someone you trust and talk about your struggle with food and weight preoccupations. If possible, share parts of this book with your friend or family member or ask the person to read the book so he or she can strongly support your efforts to overcome your eating and weight problems.

Step Nine: Redefine
Your Life

What's More Important to You Than Dieting?

"The amount of time I spent thinking about food and being upset about my body was insane."

Actress Courtney Thorne-Smith, in *U.S. Weekly*[1]

"More devastating, perhaps, than the physical harm I was doing to myself, and I could not stop doing, was the psychological toll it took on me, because all the things I should have been thinking about as a thirteen-year-old girl— adventure, what I was going to be when I grew up, my schoolwork, boys, travel, who I was, what the world was, what awaited me in the world— all those things were supplanted by thoughts about food. I dreamt about food. My entire consciousness was taken up by food."

Author Naomi Wolf, testifying before Congress
about eating disorders[2]

FOR YEARS, WORRIES about my weight clouded every moment and every activity. Thinking about my body size became my hobby, my avocation, and my obsession. I spent hours each day counting calories or carbohydrates, weighing food portions, and planning what I could and couldn't eat. I read diet books and shopped for diet pills. I woke up thinking about dieting and went to sleep performing a calorie inventory for the day.

I hated dieting, and the feelings of deprivation and unsatiated hunger that I suffered, but my constant worrying filled each day with a distorted sense of purpose. I had clear goals: to lose another dress size, drop another ten pounds, or trim another inch off my hips. While I didn't consciously use dieting as a means of avoiding vulnerability and risk, I could and did frequently postpone new experiences or relationships with the magic chant "I'll do that when I'm thin enough." Although I was lonely and hurting, I believed that my quest to attain the ideal body took priority over relationships or life experiences.

When I began to live without dieting and learned to accept myself, I realized just how small and stifling my universe had become. For years I'd told myself, "When I lose weight, I'll be happy/successful/satisfied." Now, as I stopped putting my life on hold and opened myself up to new activities, I faced the challenge of looking at my life without the buffer of weight preoccupation. As I did, I began to answer the questions "Who am I?" and "What's important to me?" and "What do I want to do with each precious day of my life?"

Gradually, like a prisoner freed after years of incarceration, I started to reconnect with and rejoice in the world around me. I bought a pair of in-line skates, and a friend gave me skating lessons. I joined Amnesty International and reached out to groups working to help the mentally ill in my own community. Each day I focused less on my body and my weight and more on rediscovering my interests and values.

As I look back on this time, I realize that in opening my mind and heart to the world, I also opened the door to achieving a fit and attractive body. When I turned away from the scale and involved myself in joyful and valuable activities, a remarkable thing happened: I began to lose weight and inches without even trying. Why? Because I regained a true sense of self-worth, making it easier for me to identify and satisfy my needs—and because I filled my life with activities more interesting and rewarding than dieting or bingeing.

It's a story that I hear frequently: When men and women begin to focus on goals and interests more important than dieting, they begin to lose weight more easily. One friend of mine dieted constantly but could never lose weight until she gave birth to a child with a severe disability. Suddenly her life was filled with more crucial jobs than counting calories: she had to learn sign language, join advocacy groups, chair fund-raisers for her child's school, and spend hours each day teaching her daughter basic life skills. "I don't think I even noticed the last fifteen pounds coming off," she says. "There was so much else going on in my life that mattered more."

Dieting as a Narcissistic Act

As I learned to see myself as a nondieter, I gradually realized how much of my time I'd spent thinking about my body and my eating. I've talked about the self-loathing that accompanies dieting, but the flip side is that dieting makes us self-involved. Obsessed with our weight and our measurements— or often, in the case of men, with the size and definition of our muscles— we place enormous importance on our physical appearance while ignoring far more important aspects of our lives and our relationships with our world.

Recently I read an interview in which a male dieter and bodybuilder told a *48 Hours* reporter, "You're obsessed with every tiny body part. You want to make sure every little cut is there, every little muscle group is defined. . . . I can never see a day where I can look in the mirror and say, 'Oh, you know, I'm 100 percent; I'm perfect.'"

That comment strikes me as terribly sad and shallow at this point in my life. Doesn't this young, healthy, intelligent person have anything more valuable to do with his energy, time, and money than worry about the definition of his muscle groups? When he looks in the mirror, does he see a human being behind the image or just a chunk of tissue to be molded into a "perfect" shape?

Yet how different was that remark from my own attitude fifteen years earlier? I can remember when achieving physical "perfection" was far more important to me than the well-being of my neighborhood, my community, or my world—and I can remember basing my self-worth less on my personal characteristics than on my success in pursuing an unrealistic, unhealthy, and narrow definition of beauty. For years I put my life in a holding pattern, divorcing myself from the world because of my perceived physical imperfections. Like the bodybuilder obsessed with sculpting each muscle, I spent much of my life believing that my body mattered more than anything else in the world.

It's a tragically narrow perception, but one that millions of people share: surveys show that 15 percent of women and many men would trade five years of their life simply to be thin.

Magazine ads often promise that the right diet plan, pound-evaporating herb, or weight-loss pill can "change your life forever." Why do we buy wholeheartedly into such a promise? Because a defining mindset of chronic dieters is that we view our body size as more important and our envisioned weight loss as more life-altering than even our greatest achievements.

During the time that being thin became my criterion for self-acceptance, I completed college and was accepted into medical school. But making good grades in demanding classes wasn't as big an achievement, in my mind, as losing ten pounds or dropping a dress size. During the same time, famine wracked Africa, East Germany opened the Berlin Wall, Rock Hudson became the first major American celebrity to die of AIDS . . . and Karen Carpenter became the first major American celebrity to die from anorexia. Yet I remained disconnected from it all. It was meaningless, compared to my preoccupation with achieving a perfect figure.

Clearly I'd internalized the message of the national weight-loss program that once made women who didn't meet their weight goals sing, "We are plump little pigs . . . fat and forlorn." No matter what I did, how many lives I touched, or how much knowledge I gained, I saw myself as that pig, forlorn, unlovable, and an object of ridicule—and I saw my struggle to lose weight as the most important event in my life. If I'd magically been given a chance to trade five years of my own life for a permanent loss of twenty pounds, I would have done it—instantly.

Why do we become so obsessed with our bodies that we value them more than our minds, our spirits, our accomplishments, our very lives, and the world around us? I've already discussed how the media train us to worry constantly about our looks and our size. But another reason for our body obsession, in my opinion, is the shrinking of our "village" of friends and family.

A friend of mine, recently returned from Europe, commented on the sense of community she found there. At Greek parties teenagers danced with their grandparents, and entire families shared stories and singing. In France, girls walked hand-in-hand to school.

Americans, in contrast, place paramount importance on the nuclear family. Most of us know little or nothing about the people who live across the street from us, the people with whom we shop or work, or even our aunts, uncles, cousins, nieces, and nephews. We lead lives more "separate" than earlier generations, or our peers in other countries—an aloneness exacerbated by the fact that even our nuclear families frequently break apart.

One result is that as our circle of friends and family narrows, we focus more on ourselves. And since our culture teaches us that the most important aspect of our lives is our body shape, we naturally become more and more obsessed with losing pounds and shaping muscles. This focus robs our lives of meaning and purpose, and—ironically—drives us deeper into the diet mentality that causes us to gain, not lose, weight.

Rediscovering Your Interests and Values

As you free yourself from dieting and develop a relaxed attitude toward food, you're likely to recognize the effects of "dieting narcissism" on your life. You may find it difficult to identify with friends whose primary interests are dieting, or honing their muscles at the gym. And you may detect a void in your life—a void that your preoccupation with calories or carbs, and your constant crises with starving and eating, once filled.

If you do, ask yourself an important question: Is this void, even if it causes you anxiety or sadness, a positive sign of change? The empty feeling that you once masked with dieting or overeating may be your soul crying out for meaning in your life: for healthy relationships, new experiences and opportunities, new challenges to face. If so, it's crucial to confront and even welcome this feeling, rather than retreating back to a bag of potato chips or another diet. Facing and filling the empty spaces in our lives takes concentration and work—work that we too often avoid by turning to food for comfort or focusing on weight as the root of all of our problems. Becoming aware of your feelings and acting on your awareness is a necessary step toward freeing yourself from this cycle.

Can you reframe your perception, perceiving your boredom or emptiness not as a sign of failure but as an opportunity to fill the void in your life by rediscovering your interests and talents? If so, the next step is to identify the aspects of your life that need work. To begin, ask yourself the following questions.

Do I Need New and Better Relationships?

All too frequently we involve ourselves in harmful relationships or avoid seeking healthy ones. Confronting our reasons for doing this can be painful: Do we accept cruel or weak partners because we think little of ourselves? Do we avoid serious relationships because we're fearful of being rejected, wounded, or let down? Do we let our friends or family members mistreat us because we unconsciously accept the role of martyr?

Answering these questions requires looking into our souls and making an active commitment to connect with our deepest feelings. It's far easier to curl up in front of the TV, nurse our wounds, and reach for a carton of Ben and Jerry's or a can of Pringles—or to postpone the hard work of creating healthy relationships by saying "Dieting will solve all of my problems. I'll find someone who treats me better when I'm a size 8."

When my life stopped revolving around dieting and body preoccupations, I had to learn to do without these crutches and face problem relationships head-on. At first it was difficult. But as I became more honest about my needs and my self-worth, I gained the strength to break off unsatisfying relationships and to seek out male and female friends who treated me well. And I learned to say to others, "This is who I am. I am worthy of your love and respect."

If you feel bored, stifled, or oppressed by your relationships, now is the time for you to take this step. Stop telling yourself that "someday" you'll seek out rewarding relationships. Decide that "someday" is today.

What New Experiences and Knowledge Do I Want to Gain?

Did you always want to take up painting? Learn to play the piano? Climb mountains? Master a foreign language? Then take the time, energy, and money you once spent on dieting, bingeing, and food obsession and redirect those resources toward learning and growing. As you do, you'll see the difference between the joy you gain from true accomplishment and the brief "high" you gain from the false accomplishment of temporarily losing a few pounds.

Here's an exercise that will encourage you in your resolve to grow as a person as you replace dieting with more important and interesting activities:

1. In your journal, make a list of five new skills you'd love to learn and five experiences you hope to have during your lifetime.

2. List what you need to be able to enjoy these experiences or learn these new skills. For instance: Will you need money? A baby-sitter for your children, so you can travel? Help from your partner, so you can go back to school?

3. Make it your goal to fulfill at least one of the dreams on your list within the year—or, if the dream is big, to take an active step toward fulfilling it. (For instance, if you've always wanted to visit a foreign country or take a cruise, start a travel fund.)

4. Calculate how much money you typically spend each year on diet programs, diet books, diet pills, and other weight-loss products. Now that you're not dieting, this is "free" money! If accomplishing your dreams requires money, get an empty jar from your pantry and start putting your nondiet money in the jar each month. If you're like most dieters, you'll wind up, in a year or two, with several hundred dollars in your jar—enough to fund a small adventure or start a nest egg for a larger one.

As you accomplish each goal or enjoy each experience, add another to your list of want-to-dos. It doesn't matter if your goals are big (to go to law school) or small (to see a show on Broadway or learn to make puff pastry). What matters is that you expand your horizons and stretch yourself in ways that define who you are and what you enjoy, now that dieting is no longer the center of your life.

What Can I Do to Make a Difference in the World?

Of all the actions I ask you take in this step, this is the most important. In the previous steps I asked you to know yourself, respect yourself, and concentrate on yourself to achieve long-term weight loss. Now I'm asking you to do just the opposite: to look at the world around you and to ask yourself what you can do for others.

Dieting makes us focus obsessively on our own bodies and our own suffering. Moreover, it demands our time, energy, and money, often keeping us from using our resources to make a difference in the lives of those around us. Who has time to build houses for Habitat for Humanity when we're spending hours at the gym defining our muscles or locked in our rooms, starving or bingeing? In our pursuit of unrealistic beauty ideals, we often become lit-

tle more than "meat puppets," with small purpose to our lives beyond looking buff or Barbie-ish. In doing so, we deprive ourselves of one of the greatest gifts of life: the ability to make the world better, in large ways or small,
than it would be without us.

To gain some insight into the difference between shallow goals based on
"look-ism" and real life goals that give your life meaning, take this quick test.

On a sheet of paper, list five people you admire for their contributions to the
world—for instance, Albert Schweitzer, Rosa Parks, Paul Newman, Lech Walesa,
Oprah Winfrey, or even the unknown young man who faced down the tanks in
Tiennamen Square. It doesn't matter if the person is famous; if you like, list members of your own family.

Next, under each person's name, answer the following questions:

1. Do you admire this person solely because of his or her looks or for
   other reasons?
2. Is this person important to the world because he or she is or was thin
   or well muscled?
3. If you wrote this person's epitaph, what would it say?

Examine your answers. Did you write that your hero was important because
"She was a size 6," or "He had well-defined abs"? Or did you say, "He saved lives,"
"She sent a message to African-American women that they could succeed," "She
stood up for freedom," "He helped people less fortunate than himself," "He risked
his life to make his country a better place for the next generation"?

Now, do the same activity, only list your name.

What would you want the world to remember you for? If no one could think
of anything to say on your tombstone other than "She lost some cellulite on her
hips" or "He increased his chest size by two inches," would you feel that your life
had served a purpose? If not, what would you rather be remembered for?

Most likely your list will reveal that the people you admire come in many
different sizes and shapes and their lives were important not because they
looked like MTV stars but because they wanted their existence to mean
something. Like them, you can make a difference to your world—but you

won't do it by obsessing about the calorie content of your tuna fish or the number of reps you did today at the gym.

Instead, look inside yourself and ask yourself, "What problems do I see around me? What skills do I have that could help to solve these problems?" Do you have a particular interest in protecting the environment or preserving historical sites in your neighborhood or promoting research on diabetes? If so, find a way to contribute to these causes.

If you're busy, you can contribute to the world in small but meaningful ways—for instance, by adopting a pet from the pound, donating blood, or cleaning out your pantry and donating cans of food to the nearest food bank. If your life seems empty and you have unfilled hours, on the other hand, think about volunteering at a hospital or nursing home, being a Special Olympics coach, or signing up as a Big Brother or Big Sister.

When you do, you'll accomplish four goals. First, you'll make your own life more meaningful. Second, you'll make a real difference to the world—far more of a difference than if you spent the same effort jogging on a treadmill, or counting the fat grams in your Healthy Choice lasagna. Third, your volunteer efforts will open your eyes to how petty America's focus on weight and body image is, when real and serious problems exist all around us. And fourth—believe it or not—you'll lose your excess pounds more easily.

Surprise! Why *Not* Thinking About Weight Makes You Lose Weight

Here's another great reason to get off your scales and get out into the world: you'll actually lose weight faster, and keep it off more successfully, if you stop obsessing about it. Really! There's a good reason for this phenomenon. When you're busy tutoring inner-city children in math, or visiting your grandmother at the nursing home, or taking piano lessons, your mind isn't obsessing about food. Instead, the empty time you once filled with food is filled with productive work, physical activity, new friends, and new opportunities for fun, achievement, and self-esteem.

Moreover, focusing on goals more important than weight loss helps you to cope with the fact that real weight loss, the kind that's permanent and healthy, takes time (see Step Seven). People who step on the scale three times a day are far more likely to become discouraged and binge than people who are so busy with meaningful activities that they forget to worry about weight.

Terry Poulton, author of No Fat Chicks, *battled weight for most of her life, trying diet after diet. In the 1980s, she subjected herself to a high-profile diet sponsored by the women's magazine* Chatelaine, *which celebrated her weight loss by putting her on the cover. But you can guess the story: she quickly regained the weight she'd lost, and suffered the humiliation of being a public "diet failure."*

Eventually, Poulton rejected the tyranny of cultural expectations and became a crusader for women's rights—including the right to have a healthy body, not starved into an unnatural state. Helping other women escape the trap of dieting became her new goal, and she completely stopped dieting and worrying about her weight.

Ironically, she notes, "I have found to my delight and amazement after a lifetime of fighting my weight every step of the way that when my mental attitude was finally healed, my body automatically began sorting itself out." When she ate what and when she wished, she lost approximately fifty pounds. (I say "approximately" because Poulton no longer owns a scale.) "I don't look like Kate Moss or Twiggy," she says, "and I never will. . . . But with a reasonable amount of steady effort—which I now want to make, for my health and my appearance—I am working on achieving the best possible version of my own natural physique."

Poulton is pleased about her weight loss, but if you ask her what's more important—her weight, or the tremendous positive impact she's had on other women trying to break free from cultural stereotypes—I'm sure she'll say it's the latter. The weight loss, while it's a predictable result of focusing her energies on bettering her world rather than on counting calories and carbohydrates, is just icing on the cake.

It's our worst nightmare, as dieters, that if we stop dieting and spend our time and energy doing something else, we will turn into human blimps. We are convinced that if we're stripped of our obsession with "good" and "bad" foods, we will lose all control over our bodies, becoming huge and unattractive. But the exact opposite is true: When weight stops ruling our lives, the pounds come off more easily. It is *dieting itself* that makes us overweight, and when we abandon dieting (and the impossible goal of looking like starved models) and turn our lives to more important and meaningful pursuits, we actually make our bodies more beautiful.

So make it your mission to find meaning in your life—whether it's by reconnecting with family members, volunteering at the local food bank (nothing points out the foolishness of food obsession better than meeting people who have no food!), or expanding your mind by taking up new activities. When you do, you'll be surprised at how joyous life can be when you're not consumed with thoughts about weight, and how much more easily the pounds melt away when you make your life count for something instead of simply counting calories. It's one of the remarkable paradoxes of life—enjoy it!

Step Ten: Give to the Next Generation

Preventing Eating Disorders and Obesity in Children

"The best way to lift one's self up is to help some one else."

Booker T. Washington[1]

WHEN YOU COMPLETE the first nine steps of this program, you'll be on the path to a lifetime of health, fitness, and freedom from weight problems. But there's one more crucial step you can take—not for yourself but for the sake of the children who follow in your footsteps.

As a parent, teacher, friend, or relative of young children, you can teach the next generation to grow up proud of themselves and their bodies. You can help them avoid obesity and immunize them against the diseases of compulsive dieting, bulimia, and anorexia. You can teach them to recognize and reject the cultural stereotypes that lead to poor health, chronic dieting, and low self-esteem and to savor and appreciate food without fear or guilt.

You and I can't change the powerful forces of our culture overnight. But each of us *is* strong enough to refuse to let that culture destroy the individual children we care about—and each child we save from food and body preoccupations will be one less life ruined by obesity, eating disorders, debilitating body preoccupation, and self-loathing.

The Epidemic of Childhood Obesity and Eating Disorders

How many American children suffer the devastating effects of our culture's conflicting messages about weight and food? One index is the massive and increasing number of overweight children. More than a fifth of American children are overweight, obese, or extremely obese, an increase of 50 percent since 1960,[2] and our kids are becoming overweight at ever-younger ages.

This epidemic stems from a sad cycle, repeated in millions of households across America. Our children put on excess pounds, often because of a steady diet of junk food, television, and video games, combined with the stresses of modern life—or sometimes they merely put on a few pounds of "baby fat" as a normal and healthy result of aging and puberty. We respond by doing exactly what the doctors tell us to do: sending our children to diet programs and diet camps, counting their calories and carbohydrates, and scolding them for eating "bad" foods. Our children try their hardest to stick to these diets—because they know the harsh penalties for being overweight in America as well as we do—but eventually they begin bingeing or overeating, often shamefully and secretively. As a result they grow more and more overweight, becoming increasingly unpopular with peers who judge their worth by their body size. They endure constant bullying, verbal abuse, shunning, and daily victimization by children and adults taught by our culture that it's OK to ridicule or even hate overweight people. They turn to food for comfort, magnifying their weight and self-esteem problems and beginning a downward spiral that may last a lifetime.

In short, in our efforts to help our children we instead set them up for exactly the same patterns of yo-yo dieting, bingeing, overeating, lifetime weight gain, and humiliation that cause us so much pain.

But there are even worse consequences: in addition to the terrible stigma of being overweight in a fat-phobic culture, overweight children risk developing serious medical problems. Physicians now see frightening numbers of young children with type 2 diabetes, a disease once diagnosed almost exclusively in adults, and according to endocrinologist Kenneth Lee Jones, "The wave of this is just beginning to break."[3] The cause of this crisis is the rising number of overweight children and teens, and the price these young diabetics will pay may be a terrible one (see sidebar). Yet the only tool most doctors offer to prevent this tragedy is dieting—an approach that's generally as ineffective for children as for adults.

A "Middle-Age" Disease Strikes the Young

Type 1 diabetes, caused by destruction of insulin-producing pancreatic cells, usually strikes in childhood. In contrast, type 2 diabetes, in which the body produces insulin but doesn't use it efficiently, generally occurs in people over age forty-five. (In fact, doctors once referred to type 2 diabetes as *adult-onset diabetes*.) But this "grown-up" disease now afflicts thousands of young adults, teens, and even preteens.

Serious complications of type 2 diabetes typically set in fifteen to twenty years after onset, meaning that diabetic children could begin to suffer devastating problems including kidney failure, limb loss, heart disease, or blindness in their twenties or thirties. Moreover, the American Diabetes Association warns, "There is already mounting evidence that type 2 diabetes may be more aggressive when it occurs at a young age."[4]

If your child is significantly overweight, and particularly if type 2 diabetes runs in your family, ask your physician if your child should be tested for diabetes. African-American, Hispanic, and Native American children are at highest risk for childhood diabetes. Children with type 2 diabetes generally take oral medication rather than requiring insulin shots, and several newer drugs for type 2 diabetes can also help diabetic children lose weight.

Sadly, diets—the only preventive treatment generally offered by doctors—are of little use in *preventing* childhood obesity and resulting diabetes. However, a child who is diagnosed as diabetic will need to follow dietary rules to keep his or her blood sugar from reaching dangerous levels.

While many children struggle with obesity, many others—most of whom aren't even overweight—buy into the myth that they can (and must) diet their way to model-thin bodies. Little girls are dieting in record numbers, and a recent survey reported that 36 percent of third-grade boys have tried to lose weight.[5] In a recent issue of the *Chicago Sun-Times*, physician Ira Sacker described a *six-year-old* who ate paper to curb her hunger, because she so feared gaining weight. "These aren't isolated cases anymore," he said. "It seems to be a trend."[6]

What starts as dieting in elementary school frequently becomes an eating disorder in high school and college. These diseases are now so common that students complain that school bathrooms reek from the vomit of bulimics, and almost every student knows someone with severe anorexia.

Awash in media images that promote artificial thinness while relentlessly hawking high-calorie, high-fat, sugary fast foods, our children lack the maturity to deal with either the pressures to diet or the temptations to overeat. Thus it's up to us, as their role models and mentors, to offer guidance. But what can you do, as an individual, to prevent a child from developing food and body image problems or to help a child who's already overweight? As a parent and a therapist, I recommend these seven simple but powerful keys.

Love Unconditionally

The parents remind me of wedding-cake models, attractive in an almost too-perfect way. She's second in line for a CEO position; he's a successful owner of a software company. They're smart, funny, and generous, the kind of people you want as your friends. Their son, too, is picture-perfect, a track star and straight-A student.

There's a daughter, too, but they don't brag about her as much. Kim gets straight As too, and she has a wry sense of humor, a talent for painting, and a fierce sense of loyalty to her friends. She also has a weight problem: at seventeen, she weighs 225 pounds.

As a slightly chubby child, Kim cringed when she sensed her parents' unspoken shame. Even though she wasn't obese until later, after years of failed diets, she already felt out of place in this model family—as though she were a moose changeling born into a family of gazelles. She started her first diet at fourteen, but each diet led to failure, and each failure made her turn, guiltily and secretively, to the comfort of overeating.

As she reached her late teens, Kim grew weary of the well-intentioned diets, the visits to doctors, and her parents' eventual descent into bribes—"We know it's hard to diet, and we want to help motivate you. So if you can spend six months on Weight Watchers, and lose at least thirty pounds, we'll buy the new bedroom set you've been saving for." It was even worse on the rare occasions when they lost their tempers: "Why do you think we're thin? We watch what we eat. We exercise. We eat broccoli even if we want cake. You could do it if you'd just try harder."

Kim went to Weight Watchers and initially lost twenty-five pounds, but within six months she'd gained back forty-five. She didn't get her bedroom set, but eventually her parents stopped asking her about her weight. "These days I just get the look," she says. It's not the look of pride her parents give her thin brother; it's a look of suppressed anger and shame. And when she sees it, she hides in her room, where she has a stash of cookies and candy bars hidden in her book bag.

As parents, we love our children desperately and deeply. But sometimes, despite our best intentions, our love comes with strings attached, and those strings can strangle a child's fragile self-esteem.

In Kim's case the condition her parents attached to their love was "You must be thin." Kim's parents' and sibling's slimness made her burden even greater. Yet baby pictures clearly showed that other family members had been slender from birth, while Kim was a somewhat chunky toddler. She wasn't born to be obese or even overweight—years of dieting and low self-esteem created that problem—but no matter how hard she tried, her genes prevented her from being reed-slender. Doomed to fail, she turned to food as an escape from her sadness and anxiety and eventually became a compulsive overeater.

Parents almost never intend to hurt their overweight children, but some fall into the trap of basing their own self-esteem on their children's appearance or achievements. Kim's parents, for instance, clearly valued the "perfect" image they projected and had difficulty accepting the "imperfection" of her body size—pushing her, ironically, from being slightly stocky to being obese. Other parents, with average-weight children, may push their sons or daughters to lose weight so these children can achieve at gymnastics, modeling, or acting, activities that place an inordinate emphasis on body size. And many overweight parents, tormented by the idea that their children will suffer the bullying and rejection that they suffered, translate this concern into an insistence on dieting and slimness. But children don't always recognize the love behind their parents' obsession with weight; what they recognize is disappointment and disapproval.

If your own relationship with your child is affected by your concerns about his or her size, and weight is becoming a major issue, ask yourself:

Do I feel embarrassed by my child's weight?

Do I feel angry at my child when I see him or her overeating?

Do I believe that my child could control his or her weight simply by trying harder?

Do I sometimes feel that my child is lazy, unmotivated, undisciplined, or lacking in willpower because of his or her weight?

Am I worried that my child will repeat a family pattern of weight problems or obesity?

If the answer to any of these questions is yes, reread Step Three, on loving yourself, and then apply the same principles to every interaction with your child. While all parents and children are unique, the one nonnegotiable rule is that *your children must know that you love them exactly as they are*—and that you will love them whether they weigh 80, 180, or 480 pounds. No "We'll buy you new clothes if you can take off five pounds." No "Maybe you could exercise more, like your sister does." No "Why don't you stand in the back there behind Tim, so your hips won't show in the picture?" No outpouring of attention and rewards if your child does lose weight, a response that can teach your child that your love is conditional.

Instead, let your child know without any doubt whatsoever that your love won't increase or decrease depending on the number on the bathroom scale. Cherish the gift of your child's presence in your life each day and show it. Be sure you give hugs and kisses on a regular basis and take time to cuddle your child. *To be fit, your child must first love him- or herself—and have your unconditional love as well.*

Also, recognize that becoming fit can be difficult for children because of a host of reasons ranging from genes to school tensions and that a child who's overweight isn't lazy, low on willpower, or weak, but rather is courageously coping in an openly hostile world (see sidebar on page 192). Admire your child for doing this and do everything you can to make the experience easier—not harder.

I do want to make it very clear that even if you do love your child unconditionally, he or she may develop a weight problem or an eating disorder. These problems have multiple emotional and biological roots, and many are beyond your control as a parent, so there is no reason to feel guilty if you (like millions of other American parents) are dealing with children's weight issues. But you can lower the risk of your child's developing serious lifelong weight problems or dangerous eating disorders, as well as facilitate your child's efforts to overcome any of these problems, by loving without reservation.

Foster Healthy Attitudes About Food

Today's children are caught in a double bind: the media saturate them with commercials for sugar- and fat-laden foods and at the same time tell them that they must be unnaturally thin to find love and success. Add to this the "wired" lifestyle of many children, who spend hours each day watching TV, playing computer games, and talking on cell phones, instead of climbing trees and riding bikes, and you have a prescription for both obesity and eating disorders.

Under these conditions parents can't simply assume that children can learn healthy attitudes about eating and health. Instead we must actively teach them, without being judgmental or moralistic. Here are my recommendations for promoting healthy eating habits from an early age.

Eat in the Kitchen and Dining Room

Treat food with respect and make an occasion out of meals. Use nice plates, have your children help set the table and prepare the food, and try to get your entire family to eat together as often as possible. Make it a point to put your food on plates or in bowls rather than eating out of pans or "grazing" as you walk around the house. (As author and ex-dieter Geneen Roth says, "If you eat at the refrigerator, pull up a chair"—in other words, sit down and pay attention to what you're eating and teach your children to do the same.)

Also, avoid eating in the car on a regular basis and turn off the television at snack times and meal times. Children who constantly grab meals on the run or eat continuously and almost subconsciously while watching TV put

The Bravery of Overweight Children

From an early age, overweight children learn just how brutal cultural expectations can be. Studies show that larger children are far more likely to be bullied than slim children, that even preschoolers have negative attitudes toward overweight people, and that elementary school children describe overweight peers as lazy, dirty, sloppy, ugly, and stupid.

What is remarkable is that overweight children have the courage to get up each morning and face this savage prejudice. Psychologist Michael I. Loewy says, "Fat children should be admired because being fat in our society takes tremendous strength. For fat children to face teasing, rejection, and discrimination on a daily basis and still thrive takes great strength of character."[7] Not all heroes are fighter pilots or soldiers; many of them are the little boys in husky pants and the girls in plus-size dresses who we see walking to school every day.

on more pounds than children in homes with established eating routines. In addition, they learn the unhealthy habit of using food to compensate for boredom, loneliness, or restlessness. Conversely, kids who eat at the table tend not to overeat, because when they become full, they get bored and want to get back to other activities.

I recommend starting the "eat in the kitchen/dining room" rule early, so it becomes an ingrained habit. Rather than letting a three-year-old run around the house with a sippy cup of juice or sit in front of the TV with a box of crackers, for instance, turn off the cartoons and have your child sit at the table when it's snack time.

Another tip: don't encourage "eating out of the bag," which fosters unconscious eating. Instead of cringing if your child asks for potato chips, say "Sure! Turn off the TV, come into the kitchen, and I'll give you a bowl." (If your child says a bowlful isn't enough, simply respond that more is available if he or she is still hungry when the first bowl is empty.)

Avoid Making a Habit of Rewarding Your Child with Food

It's fine to occasionally say "You've really worked hard practicing for the recital; let's go grab an ice cream cone." But also make a point of rewarding your child with other, nonfood activities such as a trip to the park, extra mall money, or a game of basketball in the backyard. This will teach your child to find comfort and satisfaction in a range of pleasures including, but not limited to, food.

Be a Role Model

Rather than nagging about food and weight, set an example by living a healthy lifestyle yourself. For instance, if you don't want to encourage your child to wolf down food in front of the TV, avoid doing so yourself. If you make a rule that your child must eat in the kitchen or dining room, sitting down at the table, be sure you follow this rule yourself.

More important, show your child that you enjoy eating without worrying unhealthily about food or body issues. Do you find yourself making comments such as "I really shouldn't eat this" or "I feel so sinful having another cookie" or "I'll pay for this later"? Instead, focus on making positive comments about eating—for instance, "Isn't this steak that Dad cooked delicious?" or "I'm really enjoying this fresh asparagus, aren't you?"

By treating eating as natural and pleasurable, you'll greatly reduce your child's risk of obesity and eating disorders. John Reilly and colleagues at Glasgow Royal Hospital for Sick Children surveyed a hundred children and found that "over-anxious parents who are concerned that their children will develop problematic eating habits might actually be encouraging this sort of pattern to develop." The researchers found that children as young as five are developing unhealthy preoccupations about eating and weight that put them at risk for disturbed eating behavior.[8]

Buy the Foods Your Child Likes

This is critical. Even if your child is overweight, do *not* make lists of "forbidden" foods that can't be brought into your home. (The only exception is if your child has a medical condition, such as diabetes or an allergy to peanuts, that requires certain foods to be limited or avoided.)

That doesn't mean that you need to buy *every* food your child desires. Instead let your child choose one or two grocery items each week, without being judgmental about whether these foods are "healthy" or not. In this way you'll limit the supply of cookies, candy, and chips in your house, not by banning them but by teaching your child to make conscious choices about the foods he or she truly desires.

Prohibiting "bad" foods is a prescription for disaster, because children forbidden to eat Oreos or Fritos will become obsessed with the taboo foods and move heaven and earth to obtain them. This, in turn, can establish a lifelong pattern of guilt and secrecy. Conversely, children allowed to eat any foods they want—as long as they sit at the table, in the kitchen or dining room—often become bored with the chips, candy, and other foods they once coveted.

A recent study showed dramatically that making certain foods taboo merely teaches children to crave them. Researchers chose two snack foods that children typically like and offered both foods freely for several weeks. Then they provided unlimited amounts of one food, while placing the other in a jar and telling the children it was off-limits. Later, when the children again received permission to eat the restricted snack food, they took larger portions of it and ate more of it than they had before it was restricted.[9]

In addition, restricting a child's food intake forces the child to rely on external cues rather than on internal hunger, a prescription for obesity or eating disorders. Another group of researchers recently surveyed nearly two hundred children and their moms and found that the daughters of mothers who restricted "bad" foods ate more snack foods when they could get them, because they had a reduced ability to identify hunger and satiety cues.[10] Clearly, while you don't want to overload your pantry with less-than-healthy foods, you don't want to create an unnatural desire for these foods by banning them, either.

Katherine grew up with a mother who struggled endlessly, and unsuccessfully, to lose weight. When Katherine put on pounds as she reached puberty, her mother reacted in terror. To Katherine's shame and embarrassment, her mother even went so far as to padlock the pantry door when she left Katherine at home alone.

Not surprisingly, Katherine craved the "bad" foods she couldn't have. "When my mother and father left for a movie or dinner date," she told me, "I'd become desperate for something other than the carrot sticks and celery my mother allowed me to eat. I remember using egg whites and some sugar I scrounged up to whip together a large bowl of meringue. I would wolf down the meringue, feeling simultaneously relieved and rebellious."

Rather than restricting ice cream and other treats, keep them on hand and tell your child, "We're going to eat dinner, and then there's ice cream if you want it." (This is a better approach than saying "You can't have ice cream until you clean your plate," because the first approach tells your child that the food is readily available and that you're not exerting control over access to it while also teaching your child that the food is eaten after dinner as part of a family routine.)

Also, prepare nutritious meals, but don't get into a power struggle if your child refuses to eat your stir-fry and instead opts for peanut butter and jelly or a hamburger with friends. This doesn't mean that you need to prepare a second meal for your child. Instead, let your child know that you're enjoying your meal and that he or she can prepare another simple dish. If your child is too young to cook, explain that you'll help fix something else after you finish eating (if that's something you're willing to do). Keep it simple. Be careful to communicate to your child that you won't prepare second meals on a regular basis.

Most kids eventually decide that they like fruits, vegetables, and other healthy foods, but trying to control them won't help. A more positive way to encourage children to eat healthy foods is to involve them in cooking from an early age. The child who peels the bananas for the fruit salad or snaps the green beans all by himself often has a more positive attitude toward eating these foods. Also, offer a new food several times, without forcing it on your child; according to one expert, it takes an average of seven tries to get a child to try a new food.

I do recommend that you don't keep sodas in the house, especially if your child hasn't already been introduced to them. Kids who fill up on soda or an excess amount of juice tend to eat a smaller variety of healthy foods, as well as to have more cavities.

Educate Without Lecturing

Instead of dividing foods into "good" and "bad" categories, educate your children about what makes certain foods healthier than others. For instance, mention casually, "I like to put tomatoes on my sandwich, because they have lots of vitamins, they keep my body strong, and they taste really good." Or say, "Ice cream is fine, but Grandma likes to eat ice milk sometimes too, because it's yummy and it keeps her blood vessels healthier." Provide the knowledge your children need to make smart decisions, without turning food choices into a moral issue. I tell my kids, "Milk helps make your bones strong," and "Turkey meat helps make your muscles big."

Help Your Child Connect Eating with Hunger

At the end of a meal, tell a three- or four-year-old, "Wow, my tummy is full," or, "I feel nice and full now. I think I've had enough." If your child hasn't eaten for several hours, say, "Are you hungry? Your tummy might really enjoy a snack when you're hungry"—and afterward, say, "Are you full now? Does your tummy feel good?" Observing you as you identify hunger and satiety cues will help your children do the same.

Also, let your child leave food on the plate if he or she gets full before finishing. If you're worried about an underweight child who eats only a little at each meal, offer healthy snacks. (My younger daughter, for instance, often likes to have a banana or a glass of milk before bedtime.) When my older daughter gets full after eating a few bites, I tell her I'll save her plate in case she feels hungry later. Saying "You can't have anything to eat now, because you didn't finish your dinner," can set the stage for negative and unhealthy attitudes toward food.

Offer Real, Good-Tasting Foods

An overweight child who gets runny diet syrup with breakfast, artificially sweetened yogurt for lunch, and dry broiled chicken for dinner will probably decide, "Good food tastes horrible." Forgo the artificial sweeteners unless your family likes the taste of them and avoid buying any fat-free or sugar-free products that simply taste awful. (If they pass the taste test, they're OK.) Otherwise you may keep your child from learning to like foods that are both delicious and nutritious.

Let Your Child See Men Serving and Women Eating

As I noted earlier, one constant cultural message is "Men eat, women prepare." But you'll instill healthier attitudes about food if your children see women enjoying food and men enjoying their pleasure. If you're a man, help with the cooking and serving of food. If you're a woman, make cooking and serving a family activity—and sit down and eat with your family rather than running from stove to table to sink.

Don't Put Your Child on a Diet!

At thirteen I attended my first weight-loss program, weighing in excitedly every week. I lost weight, but not enough to make me happy; I remember being in the backyard with the other neighborhood kids, wearing shorts and feeling that my stomach was flatter but that my hips were still too wide.

When the diet program didn't make me "perfect," I tried eating only salad. Within a year I moved on to diet pills, and within a few more years I was a full-fledged bulimic.

If your child is overweight, I can almost guarantee that your pediatrician will prescribe a diet—but as a parent and a physician, I urge you to question this advice. In some cases there are valid medical reasons for children to follow restricted food plans; for instance, a diabetic child needs to avoid excess sweets and follow regular eating habits. But diets rarely lead to long-term weight loss, as the research cited in this book makes clear, and they're usually even more harmful for children than for adults. Because children's bodies are still growing, strict diets can lead to early osteoporosis[11] and stunt growth.[12] They can also precipitate depression,[13] and very-low-calorie diets can interfere with thinking and learning, especially if they reduce iron levels in girls and cause anemia.[14] Remember this key rule: in a growing child, weight *maintenance*, not weight loss, is the goal.

Moreover, all eating disorders begin with dieting, and even *moderate* dieting—the kind that most doctors mistakenly believe is safe—puts teens at risk for dangerous eating disorders. A 1999 study found that girls who go on severe diets are eighteen times more likely than other girls to develop anorexia or bulimia and that even those who go on "sensible" diets are five times more likely than nondieting girls to develop eating disorders.[15] In addition to the psychological damage done by these eating disorders, they often are deadly: one recent study followed up anorexic patients and found that two decades after diagnosis 16 percent of the patients had died from anorexia-related causes.[16] Children who become trapped in the diet mentality are also at risk for taking up smoking or using illegal drugs in a desperate attempt to take off pounds.

In short, diets probably *won't* help your child lose weight, very possibly *will* jeopardize his or her health (possibly for a lifetime), and *will* dramatically increase the risk of deadly eating disorders—not to mention creating body image problems and a warped relationship with food that can lead to lasting psychological problems. So don't ask your child's physician for any type of diet plan unless it's medically necessary. Instead, request a thorough checkup to spot any medical conditions that could contribute to your child's excess pounds. Also tell the pediatrician if your child shows signs of anxiety or depression, which can lead to overeating. If the checkup reveals that your child is healthy, I recommend following the advice in this chapter to help your child become fit naturally and healthily.

One more thing: throw out your scales or keep them where your child doesn't have to face them every day. You'll be able to tell if your child is gaining or losing weight, simply by looking. Asking a child to weigh in every day, or even once a week or once a month, places an unhealthy emphasis on weight.

Note: If your child is significantly overweight, always consult with a medical professional to determine the causes of this weight problem. A number of medical disorders (see Step Six) can cause obesity, and some affect children as well as adults. Also, if a doctor recommends dietary restrictions for valid medical reasons, be sure to follow these restrictions.

Get Fit Together

If your child is overweight, try to notice how much he or she actually *moves*. Does your daughter lie on her bed all evening, talking on the phone and watching TV? Does your son sit in front of the computer screen for three straight hours and then watch videos all night? If this is a regular pattern, take steps to make fitness a bigger part of your family lifestyle.

However, don't enforce a fitness regimen. If you do, your child will think that exercise is a punishment for being overweight. Instead, think of creative ways to involve your entire family in physical exercise. Start a tradition of family bike rides in the evenings after dinner or go on nature hikes with your children. Take up fun physical games such as Twister and badminton. Make sure your kids have bats, balls, and (if you can afford them) skateboards, roller blades, and bikes. Ask them if they'd like to join a sports team at the Y, or take tennis or swimming lessons. Put on your kids' favorite CDs and dance with them in the living room. Fitness is a habit, and if you instill that habit now, your child is likely to continue exercising into adulthood. But don't focus on the weight-reducing aspects of exercise, or make exercise sound grim. Focus instead on the fun of exercise, and how it makes people healthier and happier in general.

Also, limit your child's TV and computer time, whether your child has a weight problem or not. Again, I don't recommend an outright ban, which will merely create "TV craving." But avoid using TV as a baby-sitter when your children are little, and set a well-thought-out time limit for older kids. (Do be flexible on special occasions—for instance, if your child has a new friend over.) Research shows that children are nearly five times as likely to be overweight if they watch more than five hours of television per day than they are if they watch very little TV.[17]

Help Your Child Develop Interests, Talents, and Self-Esteem

Too often, children (like adults) use food to compensate for boredom, loneliness, a lack of meaning in their lives, or low self-esteem. Protect your children from developing this habit by helping them find out who they are, what they're interested in, and what they're good at doing. For instance:

• **Involve your child, early on, in activities that help improve his or her world.** A teen who volunteers with Habitat for Humanity, works as a hospital volunteer, or serves as a Special Olympics coach will learn that there are more important things in life than food and weight.

• **Encourage your child to try new hobbies.** A child who learns to love painting, bowling, or karate will find these activities more rewarding than sitting in front of the TV eating. But don't pressure your child to win at sports or to become an expert pianist or dancer. The last thing a sensitive child (and particularly an overweight child) needs is another reason to feel inadequate.

- **Make a point of noticing your child's strengths and pointing them out.** Children, and especially overweight children, need the self-esteem that comes with accomplishment. Every child is great at something; maybe yours has a green thumb, writes wonderful poems, or is clever at math or science. Spot these aptitudes, nurture them, and let your child know that you admire his or her special gifts. Two cautions: avoid pigeonholing your child ("Joe's the smart one, and Sarah's the athlete"), and remember that praising accomplishments should be done in addition to, not instead of, loving your child unconditionally.

Also, foster competence in your child, by encouraging independence in cooking, fix-it skills, academic skills, and other areas of life. A child who feels competent will have higher self-esteem and find the transition to adult life easier to handle, reducing the risk of eating disorders, obesity, or other destructive behaviors.

- **Validate your child's experiences and feelings.** Sometimes parents dismiss children's opinions or make all of their decisions for them. But as I discussed earlier, people who don't learn to respect and respond to their own needs and desires often turn to food as a result. So take your children's feelings and needs seriously and respond to them consistently and logically. That doesn't mean letting your child run the show; rather, it means teaching your child that his or her perspective is valued, important, and worthy of a response.

Treat your children the way you want others to treat them and the way you want them to treat themselves. If you want your children to treat themselves with respect and dignity, offer them that respect and dignity. Remember that *your children's relationships within your family become the norm by which they'll judge all future relationships.*

Also, recognize that children sometimes act out simply because they're seeking attention. At such times, avoid telling your child, "Stop whining," and instead offer a hug and say, "Come over here. Let's talk for a few minutes."

- **Teach your child the ability simply to "be."** While it's important to nurture your child's interests, don't overschedule; instead, give your child plenty of free time to read, play, or just goof off. Overscheduled children can lose the ability to enjoy unstructured time and may overeat to fill empty hours.

- **Help your child discover life's simple pleasures.** My children delight in the opportunity to lie down on blankets in the yard and stargaze with their father and me. We also teach them to enjoy music, nature, and the pleasure of their own bodies. (For instance, my younger children enjoy having their backs massaged for a few minutes before bedtime, while the teenager in our home has discovered Jacuzzis.)

Point Out Unhealthy Cultural Messages

When you watch TV or movies with your child, point out dangerous or destructive stereotypes and talk about them together. Help your child learn to analyze the messages that the media send, rather than simply absorbing them uncritically. Talk about how TV and magazines frequently promote appearance over achievement, and share information about movie stars and athletes who've struggled with and overcome eating disorders.

Also, provide your child with healthy images to compete with the unhealthy messages the media send. Encourage your son or daughter to find role models who are notable for being brave, intelligent, creative, and strong, rather than simply for being thin, pretty, or handsome. If you have a teenage girl, buy her subscriptions to *Teen Voices* and other magazines that promote self-esteem and self-sufficiency rather than pushing false beauty ideals. (And while you're at it, take a look at the magazines *you* read, because you're a powerful role model yourself.)

In addition, teach everyone in your family—both those who are coping with weight problems and those who aren't—to respect people of different sizes and shapes. For instance, if you hear your teenage son saying, "Why are you dating Gloria? She's a tub," talk to him about the devastating effects of weight prejudice. (Many children recognize the cruelty of this prejudice more readily if you explain its similarity to racism and other forms of bigotry.) In addition, educate your family members about the fact that weight problems don't stem from laziness or lack of willpower and that, in fact, dealing with obesity takes great courage. Adopt a "zero tolerance" policy toward any teasing or bullying of people who don't fit cultural stereotypes.

Make a Continuous Effort to Be a Healthy Parent

As your child's role model, you want to be happy and healthy yourself—so treat yourself well, and be sure that your family members do so too. It's all too easy (especially for women, but often for men as well) to assume the role of martyr, "doormat," or maid, but you won't help your children if you do. Instead,

The Importance of a United Front

Parents can't always agree on everything, but arbitrary and inconsistent rules and discipline can translate into stress, anxiety, and behavior problems in children, and these problems in turn can complicate food issues.

So, if possible, sit down with your spouse or partner ahead of time, when your child isn't around, and agree on (a) what your household rules are and (b) how you plan to respond when your kids have difficulty following these rules. Once you set rules, apply them consistently, and if you decide your plan isn't working, consult with your partner before changing it. Consistent, loving discipline creates far less anxiety for children than a sporadic implementation of consequences.

Also, avoid disciplining in the heat of the moment, when you're likely to be unnecessarily harsh. And, whenever possible, avoid humiliating your child by disciplining him or her in front of friends; instead, take your child aside and talk calmly about what occurred and what the consequences will be.

insist on receiving love, respect, and support from your family, and treat yourself with dignity and respect as well. This may mean occasionally saying "no" to your children so that you can take care of your own needs.

Taking your needs and feelings seriously encourages your children to do the same. It teaches them to be strong and to form healthy relationships that will nurture their spirits, rather than teaching them to accept destructive relationships that can drive them to food for solace. Moreover, children who experience their parents being content and happy are likely to be more relaxed and more likely to give themselves permission to be content and happy in their own lives.

If you're dealing with eating and body image issues that seem overwhelming (for instance, if you're anorexic or bulimic, dangerously overweight, or dealing with issues related to sexual or physical abuse), seek therapy. A good therapist can help you conquer your problems and give you new strength and new hope—and therapy can help you break family patterns of dysfunctional thinking about food and weight before these patterns can damage another generation.

There's a common saying, "The most precious gift you can give a child is your time." To that I'd add two more gifts: your wisdom and your own well-being. If there is a positive aspect to the years stolen from you by dieting or overeating, it's that you can use your new strength, knowledge, healthy attitude, and self-esteem to be a role model. By doing so, you may help save a child you love from bulimia, anorexia, or a lifetime of suffering with weight problems—and you may even save that child's life.

Transform Your Insight into a Brighter Future for Your Children

The following exercises will help you gain insight into your attitudes about food and how to teach your children healthier approaches to eating.

Family Exploration

In your journal, describe your own parents' attitudes about food, eating, weight, and body image. As you do, think about these questions:

1. How did your parents feel about their own weight?
2. How did they feel about your weight?
3. Did they do or say anything that you feel harmed you?

Analyze what you've written and see if you spot patterns that are recurring in your own relationship with your child.

Chats with Your Child

Pay attention to the frequency with which topics involving food and weight come up in your conversations with your child during the course of a week. How many of your comments were positive or neutral? How many were critical? If you detect many negative interactions, plan ways to change your "negative scripts" into positive ones.

Kids Can Cook Too

Help your child choose a favorite family recipe or a fun new recipe and enjoy preparing the food together and sharing it afterward. (Even a young child can help stir muffin batter or decorate cookies, while a teenager may enjoy planning and preparing an entire meal with you.) Cooking together helps teach your child that food is a natural and enjoyable part of life and can make your child more aware of the foods he or she eats.

Exploration of Activities

Identify other activities that your child likes and that you can enjoy together—for instance, playing basketball, dancing, or making crafts. Make these shared times a priority in your life and use them to stay in touch with what interests, excites, or concerns your child. The better your lines of communication, the more effectively your child will be able to cope with the stresses and challenges of life in a healthy, adaptive manner.

Questions I'm Often Asked

I'm thirty pounds overweight, and I know that my current weight isn't healthy. I also know that dieting doesn't work and that I need to try something new. But with all the nutrition news in the paper, I feel guilty if I eat junk food instead of good food. Isn't it better to restrict myself to foods that are healthy?

The danger in creating mental lists of "good" and "bad" foods is that you still want the "bad" foods. Eventually you may crave them so strongly that you'll break through the mental barrier you've created and experience dissociation (see Step Four). When this occurs, you disconnect from your thoughts and feelings, becoming less aware of yourself and less able to track your hunger. As a result you'll eat large amounts of the very foods you're trying to avoid.

Moreover, you may set yourself up for future episodes of overeating. When you experience dissociation, you experience euphoria and a release of anxiety—somewhat comparable to a drug "rush"—that become coupled in your mind with the experience of eating. Eventually it's not just eating forbidden foods that you crave but also the "high" that comes from dissociation.

The best way to prevent episodes of dissociated eating is simply to *avoid erecting mental barriers in the first place.* As you eat the foods you enjoy, without categorizing them as "good" or "bad," you'll rediscover your ability to experience satiation. And as you experience this satiation again and again, you will reduce your calorie intake in a gradual and healthy manner while simultaneously correcting your metabolism as it recovers from the fat-conserving "starvation mode" triggered by dieting. You'll also find yourself selecting healthy foods more and more often, not as a result of guilt or self-denial but because you really want to.

Your body is programmed for self-preservation, and if you listen to it, rather than overriding its messages with artificial diets, it will send you the right signals. Trust it.

In ten years I dieted my way from a size 14 to a size 18, so I know that diets don't work! But I'm terrified to start eating normally, because when I blow my diet I always "zone out" and eat too much. For instance, I'll eat a whole bag of potato chips or crackers at a time. Won't I gain weight if I'm surrounded by fattening foods and can't control myself?

No. In the first place, you won't always crave junk food insatiably when it stops being forbidden. Did you ever desperately covet a new necklace or sweater, only to finally receive it as a gift? Most likely you wore it frequently at first, and then it simply became part of your collection—still enjoyed but no longer an object of intense desire. Similarly, once you give yourself permission to eat any foods you want, when you are truly hungry for them— and once you learn to identify your satiation and to remind yourself that the foods you love will be available to you in the future—the foods you now crave will lose their all-consuming grip on you, and you will no longer be driven to eat them to excess. You'll also stop setting yourself up for a pattern of dissociated eating (see the preceding question).

In addition, you'll rediscover how very good it feels to eat when you're hungry and to eat what you're really hungry for. There is no comparison between this feeling and the feeling you have when you zone out and eat unconsciously.

Moreover, when you follow my plan, you'll become aware of your needs, desires, and physical sensations—and it is ignoring these feelings, rather than acknowledging them, that causes you to zone out. Concentrating on yourself and your needs and desires takes discipline, but it's a crucial key to becoming fit for life.

If you decide to eat potato chips, for instance, concentrating on yourself means being aware of your mental state while you eat. It means learning *not* to detach from the world around you, or your own feelings, through the act of eating. Instead, as you eat each chip, you will savor the food, give your attention to the act of eating, and notice your body's sensations as you become full.

Becoming aware also means noticing when you're eating even though you aren't hungry and asking yourself if you're doing so because you're upset over an argument with your boss, problems with your partner or children, or other life stressors. And it means asking yourself at these times, Is there a more effective way to handle my feelings? Can I talk to my partner, go to the gym and get a massage, take a long hot bath, talk to a friend on the phone?

When you learn to eat when you are hungry, to enjoy your food, and to identify the triggers that cause you to eat when you're not hungry, you'll learn to feel satisfied by the food you eat and to recognize the physical cues that tell you that you're satiated. You'll also learn to identify those times when you're using food to hide from your feelings and to address those feelings head-on. The combination of these skills will give you complete control over what, when, and how much you eat—and complete freedom from the need to use diets to control your eating.

I have type 2 diabetes. Can I follow your plan?

If you're a diabetic, consult your physician about how to eat in a way that's healthiest for your body. Many doctors now believe that there are no "forbidden" foods for diabetics and that any food can be eaten at least occasionally, but you and your physician will need to determine the eating pattern that's healthiest for your body and keeps your blood sugar in a normal range.

As a diabetic, you'll need to become knowledgeable about nutrition, and you'll need to be more aware of your food choices than nondiabetics are. As you make food choices, however, keep this key concept in mind: you're choosing healthy foods because you value your body and want to take positive steps to maximize your health, *not* because other foods are "bad" or because you would be "bad" for eating them. Viewing healthy nutritional choices as a positive action you take out of self-love is far more beneficial than focusing on feelings of guilt or self-denial.

Also, find forms of exercise that you enjoy. (Be sure to consult with your physician before beginning or expanding your exercise program.) Exercise is crucial to controlling type 2 diabetes, but many diabetics give up on exercise because they believe it has to be grueling. Not true! Even moderate exercise can help normalize your blood sugar, so find three or four different activities you like—gardening, yoga, walking your dog, or any activity that gets you in touch with your body—and make the commitment to participate in these activities at least three or four times a week.

Now that I'm not dieting, I no longer experience the overwhelming cravings I used to have. Sometimes, however, I still find myself eating when I'm not hungry—-especially in the afternoons. I don't wind up bingeing like I used to, but I still eat more than I really want. Why do I still do this occasionally?

Often we turn to food when we're seeking comfort or distraction—for instance, if we're bored or stressed by work. Another factor is habit; we all fall into patterns of eating at certain times, even when we're not hungry.

Here's a good technique that some of my patients use to become aware of why they graze during the day. Note the times of day at which you're most likely to eat when you're not hungry and set a timer to go off at those times. At each "trigger time," ask yourself if you truly feel hungry. Do you feel a gnawing sensation in your stomach, is your concentration deteriorating, or are you feeling anxious because you haven't eaten for some time? If so, slow down, sit down, and satisfy your hunger with a snack or a meal. (I recommend always keeping some food available, so you will never become overly hungry.)

In addition to paying attention to trigger times, identify the physical locations in which you are most likely to lose your connection to yourself. Do you tend to graze in the car? While watching television? While sitting at the computer? I call these *zone-out zones,* and if you don't become aware of them, they can interfere with your goal of long-term weight loss. Take the information you discover about your personal trigger times and zone-out zones seriously. You may even want to make a vow to yourself, each time you enter these places, to remain aware of your feelings.

Affirmations that my patients find helpful at trigger times or in zone-out zones include:

"I will remain connected to myself."
"I will remain emotionally 'awake' and be aware of my needs and feelings."
"I will take my physical and emotional hunger seriously."
"I will satiate my physical hunger with the food of my choice when I am hungry."

"I will address my emotional hunger as a valid need, which I take seriously."

Also, if you find yourself experiencing the urge to graze, use this time to explore your reasons for reaching for food when you're not hungry. As you do, you may find different ways to meet your needs. For instance, if you reach for a candy bar at 3:00 P.M. each day because you're tired, you may find that a quick stretch, a nap, or a walk helps you more. If you eat at night because you're bored or lonely, recognizing this pattern may encourage you to take a night class or start a nighttime exercise routine—activities that will address your underlying feelings rather than masking them.

How can I counteract the enormous amount of brainwashing my daughter receives from the media? She's normal weight, but at thirteen she already thinks she's fat.

Fight fire with fire, by exposing her to media sources that don't promote slavish acceptance of unhealthy beauty standards (see my recommendations in Step Ten). Also, spend time with your daughter watching the shows that she likes and point out the unrealistic beauty stereotypes that these shows reinforce.

When she's old enough, give your daughter copies of books such as Naomi Wolf's *Beauty Myth: How Images of Beauty Are Used Against Women* and Carol Emery Normandi and Laurelee Roark's *Over It: A Teen's Guide to Getting Beyond Obsessions with Food and Weight.* Buy her biographies of Cathy Rigby and other celebrities who've coped with eating disorders and biographies of strong women who stood up to cultural stereotypes in general (for instance, Florence Nightingale and Rosa Parks). Introduce her to websites that teach young women to see through the stereotypes being forced on them. (In particular, I recommend bodypositive.com and about-face.org.) And be a role model yourself, by refusing to indulge in "look-ism" in any form and by being proud of and happy in your own body.

My fifteen-year-old daughter is 5'6". She weighed 135 pounds last year, but she's been dieting and she's down to about 108 pounds. I'm worried that she's anorexic, but when I try to talk to her about food or her dieting, she gets defensive and says that nothing's wrong. I've also caught her throwing her dinner in the trash when she thinks I'm not looking. What should I do?

You're very right to worry. Your daughter's excessive weight loss, secrecy and defensiveness, and the fact that she's still dieting even though she's very thin, are all signs of anorexia. Anorexia kills hundreds of women every year, and it's not a problem you can treat by yourself. You need to seek professional help, and quickly.

Be aware, however, that no matter how lovingly you approach your daughter, she's likely to deny that she has a problem and to be hostile to the idea of obtaining help. You may need to force her into treatment, which will take great courage on your part. I strongly recommend hooking up with other parents dealing with this issue; one good place to start is at somethingfishy.org, an outstanding website that offers a vast amount of information, treatment referrals listed by state and country, and online support groups. Also, contact the American Anorexia/Bulimia Association or the National Association of Anorexia Nervosa and Associated Disorders.

My son's coach told him that he's overweight, and the doctor says he's about ten pounds heavier than he should be. How do we handle this without making him self-conscious about his weight?

First, analyze the situation. Is your son really overweight, or is he simply a stocky child from a naturally stocky family? Is he healthy and active and fit, or does he spend most of his time in front of the TV or playing with his computer and very little time on his bike or playing ball? It's possible that your pediatrician and your son's coach are right, but it's also possible that they're using arbitrary and outdated weight charts to mistakenly classify a perfectly healthy child as overweight.

Whether or not your son has a weight problem, begin by giving him healthy messages about food and body image, to help protect him against the negative cultural influences he's exposed to every day. If he's overweight, provide him with information about why diets don't work and help him learn how to listen to his body's natural hunger and satiation cues.

If your son is very sedentary, put limits on his TV and video game time. (But be very careful *not* to present this as a "punishment" for being overweight; in reality, almost all teens need to have limits set on their TV, computer, and video game time, whether they're overweight or not.) Also, provide him with plenty of fun opportunities for exercise; for instance, buy him new roller blades or a nice bike. Take family walks in the evening and set an example for your son by enjoying physical activities yourself. Make mealtimes a family occasion, establish rules about eating only in the kitchen or dining room, and make plenty of healthy food available without placing arbitrary limits on the foods your son likes.

No matter what your child's size, never make weight or food an issue. The very best thing you can do for a child struggling with a weight problem is to be in his corner every day. That means no hassling ("You shouldn't be eating those chips"), no bribes or threats ("You can have a new scooter if you'll give up ice cream for two weeks"), and no guilt trips ("I'm asking you to eat low-fat foods only because I love you"). Simply model a healthy lifestyle and a relaxed, noncritical attitude toward food and weight, encourage and praise your child's interests and talents, and support him constantly and unconditionally.

You may also need to contact your son's coach privately, tell him that you are addressing your son's weight issues in your own way, and instruct him to avoid making negative comments—even if they're well intentioned.

Sometimes after I eat dinner, and I'm watching TV with my family, I want some popcorn even though I'm not hungry. Should I allow myself to eat the popcorn or wait until I'm hungry again?

When you remain aware of your hunger and develop the patience to wait until you're hungry to eat, it's far easier to lose weight. That doesn't mean, however, that you need to tell yourself, I can't have any popcorn, even though I'd love some. It means paying attention to how you feel if you decide to eat the popcorn. If you focus on your feelings of hunger and satiation, rather than zoning out and eating on autopilot, you're likely to discover that a handful or two of popcorn is plenty to satisfy you.

Remind yourself, too, that the popcorn will always be available and that when you do become hungry again, it will be there for you to eat.

Your steps sound so logical—but as a chronic dieter and grazer, I've completely lost touch with my ability to sense hunger. I'm afraid to trust my hunger, because I don't ever really feel either hungry or sated. What can I do?

The longer you diet, the harder it can be to regain your innate ability to recognize hunger signals. Begin by tossing out your mental lists of "good" and "bad" foods and by analyzing the triggers that make you eat for reasons other than hunger. Also, practice the exercises I outline in Steps Three and Four to help you get in touch with your body and the messages it sends you.

Once you've worked on these issues, try this approach. Pick a day that isn't a high-risk time for bingeing. (Avoid high-pressure days at work for instance, and if you're female, avoid the days just before your period.) Plan in advance to treat yourself on this day to the "dinner of your dreams." Shop ahead of time for the foods you want to eat, and on the day of your dinner eat a light but filling breakfast and lunch. Plan your dinner for a time when you're likely to be getting hungry again but won't be ravenous.

As you prepare your meal, be attuned to hunger cues (see Step Four) and to how your body reacts to the idea, sight, and smell of the foods you prepare, and enjoy your sense of anticipation as you fix your meal.

When you detect sensations of hunger, welcome and acknowledge them and respond by eating your delicious and fulfilling "dream dinner." As you do, be aware of your feelings as you eat and your changing physical sensations as you become full. You'll probably be surprised by your ability to detect and experience hunger and satiation once you open yourself up to these feelings rather than suppressing them.

If you continue to have difficulty knowing when you're hungry, try scheduling three regular meals and one or two small snacks each day, being aware of how you feel before, during, and after each meal. Or you may want to try another approach that one patient of mine, who'd dieted for decades, found helpful. We set up a plan in which she ate a small breakfast, ate a fulfilling lunch (which she did find satisfying), and then ate dinner only if she noticed signs of hunger. She did this for two days in a row, and by the third day she became aware of her hunger in the evening, ate a satisfying dinner, and felt full after eating a moderate amount.

This conscious effort to become aware of your own needs and desires requires discipline and commitment, because you're trained by dieting (and by bingeing or overeating, the natural consequences of dieting) to ignore your body's signals. However, listening to your body will become second nature in time, and the rewards of hearing and heeding your body's message—including the ability to eat freely and in a relaxed way, with no fear of losing control—will change your life!

AFTERWORD

IT HAS BEEN twenty-three years since I began my first diet. While the years I spent preoccupied about my weight and body surely drained me and robbed me of many opportunities for joy, I also gained much from enduring the experience.

I could be bitter over the lost joy, but I don't feel bitterness at all. Rather, as my journey progressed, a sense of meaning and purpose for my life became apparent.

Knowing the intense pain that we endure when we cannot accept ourselves makes me, I believe, a better and more empathic psychiatrist. I find that I spend a great deal of time with my patients simply helping them validate their feelings. It is a delight to observe those I work with as they discover that they feel the way they feel, and go through what they go through, not because they are bad, selfish, or want too much, but for some very important reasons.

Whatever your problems with food and your body are, they are a result of complex emotional and physical aspects of your being that are worthy of understanding and taking seriously.

It is my hope that this book, in addition to freeing you from the prison of food and body preoccupation, has left you more at peace with yourself and more able to experience the joy that is possible in each day, with yourself, with your family and friends, and in the community that surrounds you.

RESOURCES

The FOLLOWING IS a list if inspirational and entertaining resources, put together by Dr. Oliver-Pyatt and her friends and colleagues.

Books

Anderson, Bob. *Stretching* (updated edition). Bolinas, CA: Shelter Publications, 2000.

Atrens, Dale M. *Don't Diet.* New York: William Morrow and Company, 1988.

Bordo, Susan. *Unbearable Weight: Feminism, Western Culture, and the Body.* Berkeley, CA: University of California Press, 1993.

Burns, David M., M.D., *Feeling Good: The New Mood Therapy* (revised). New York: Wholecare, 1999.

Chernin, Kim. *The Obsession: Reflections on the Tyranny of Slenderness.* New York: Harper Perennial, 1994.

Fraser, Laura. *Losing It: False Hopes and Fat Profits in the Diet Industry.* New York: Penguin, 1998.

Freedman, Judy S. *Easing the Teasing: Helping Your Child Cope with Name-Calling, Ridicule, and Verbal Bullying.* Chicago: Contemporary Books, 2002.

Fromm, Erich. *The Art of Loving* (reprint). New York: Harper Collins, 2000.

Gottesman, Jane, and Penny Marshall. *Game Face: What Does a Female Athlete Look Like?* New York: Random House, 2001.

Hirschmann, Jane, and Carol H. Munter. *Overcoming Overeating.* Reading, MA: Addison-Wesley Publishing Company, 1988.

Kano, Susan. *Making Peace with Food.* New York: Perennial Library, 1989.

Moramarco, Jacques, and Rick Benzel. *The Way of Walking: Eastern Strategies for Vitality, Longevity, and Peace of Mind.* Chicago: Contemporary Books, 2000.

Normandi, Carol Emery, and Laurelee Roark. *Over It: A Teen's Guide to Getting Beyond Obsessions with Food and Weight.* Novato, CA: New World Library, 2001.

Peck, M. Scott. *The Road Less Traveled* (reprint). New York: Simon & Schuster, 1998.

Pipher, Mary. *Reviving Ophelia: Saving the Selves of Adolescent Girls.* New York: Ballantine Books, 1995.

Roth, Geneen. *Feeding the Hungry Heart: The Experience of Compulsive Eating.* Indianapolis: Bobbs-Merrill, 1982.

St. James, Elaine. *Simplify Your Life: 100 Ways to Slow Down and Enjoy the Things That Really Matter.* New York: Hyperion, 1994.

Snyder, Rachel. *365 Words of Well-Being for Women.* Chicago: Contemporary Books, 1997.

Wolf, Naomi. *The Beauty Myth: How Images of Beauty Are Used Against Women.* New York: William Morrow, 1991.

Websites

about-face.org—information about media/cultural influences on women's body image and self-esteem.

BodIcon (http://nm-server.jrn.columbia.edu/projects/masters/ bodyimage/toc.html)—a great website on culture and body image issues.

bodypositive.com—the "body disparagement free zone."

getfedup.com—Dr. Oliver-Pyatt's website to provide support, ideas, and resources as you follow the 10 Steps to lifelong fitness.

mediaandwomen.org—more information about the media's influence on women's body image and self-esteem.

newmoon.org—New Moon Publishing produces resources for girls and women to celebrate their power.

realwomenproject.com—a site that celebrates women's beauty and
wisdom.
somethingfishy.org—website providing information on eating disorders
and recovery.

Movies

Bagdad Cafe
Eating: A Very Serious Comedy About Women & Food
The Famine Within
Monsoon Wedding
Shrek (Don't dismiss this as just a kids movie. It offers a wonderful
portrayal of what it means to find true beauty.)
Sugar Baby
The Truth About Cats and Dogs

NOTES

Chapter 2

1. Dale M. Atrens, *Don't Diet* (New York: William Morrow and Company, 1988), 15–16.
2. Linda F. Golodner, "What Consumers Need vs. What Consumers Get." Presentation to the Federal Trade Commission, October 16, 1997 on behalf of the National Consumers League.
3. From a November 25, 1997, report by Pam Moore on KRON-TV (San Francisco).
4. Rudolph Leibel, Michael Rosenbaum, and Jules Hirsch, "Changes in Energy Expenditure Resulting from Altered Body Weight," *New England Journal of Medicine* 332, no. 10 (March 9, 1995), 621–28. See also: "Interview with Rudolph Leibel," *Scientific American* (August 1996).
5. I. M. Anderson, M. Parry-Billings, E. A. Newsholme, C. G. Fairburn, and P. J. Cowen, "Dieting Reduces Plasma Tryptophan and Alters Brain 5-HT Function in Women," *Psychological Medicine* 20, no. 4 (1990), 785–91. B. E. Wolfe, E. D. Metzger, and C. Stollar, "The Effects of Dieting on Plasma Tryptophan Concentration and Food Intake in Healthy Women," *Physiological Behavior* 61, no. 4 (April 1997), 537–41. A. E. Walsh, A. D. Oldman, M. Franklin, C. G. Fairburn, and P. J. Cowen, "Dieting Decreases Plasma Tryptophan and Increases the Pro-

lactin Response to D-Fenfluramine in Women but Not Men," *Journal of Affective Disorders* 33, no. 2 (February 21, 1995), 89–97.

6. K. D. Brownell and J. Rodin, "Medical, Metabolic, and Psychological Effects of Weight Cycling," *Archives of Internal Medicine* 154, no. 12 (June 27, 1994), 1325–30.

7. M. B. Olson, S. F. Kelsey, V. Bittner, S. E. Reis, N. Reichek, E. M. Handberg, and C. N. Merz, "Weight Cycling and High-Density Lipoprotein Cholesterol in Women: Evidence of an Adverse Effect," *Journal of the American College of Cardiology* 36, no. 5 (November 2000), 1565–71.

8. M. M. Sea, W. P. Fong, Y. Huang, and Z. Y. Chen, "Weight Cycling–Induced Alteration in Fatty Acid Metabolism," *American Journal of Physiology—Regulatory, Integrative, and Comparative Physiology* 279, no. 3 (September 2000), R1145–55.

9. Research by Hamm et al., cited in D. M. Garner and S. C. Wolley, "Confronting the Failure of Behavioral and Dietary Treatments for Obesity," *Clinical Psychology Review* 11 (1991), 729–80.

10. H. E. Meyer, A. Tverdal, R. Selmer, "Weight Variability, Weight Change and the Incidence of Hip Fracture: A Prospective Study of 39,000 Middle-Aged Norwegians," *Osteoporosis International* 8, no. 4 (1998), 373–78. M. Fogelholm, H. Sievanen, A. Heinonen, M. Virtanen, K. Uusi-Rasi, M. Pasanen, and I. Vuori, "Association Between Weight Cycling History and Bone Mineral Density in Premenopausal Women," *Osteoporosis International* 7, no. 4 (1997), 354–58.

11. S. Syngal, E. H. Coakley, W. C. Willett, T. Byers, D. F. Williamson, and G. A. Colditz, "Long-Term Weight Patterns and Risk for Cholecystectomy in Women," *Annals of Internal Medicine* 130, no. 6 (March 1999), 471–77.

12. C. J. Field, R. Gougeon, and E. B. Marliss, "Changes in Circulating Leukocytes and Mitogen Responses During Very-Low-Energy All-Protein Reducing Diets," *American Journal of Clinical Nutrition* 54, no. 1 (July 1991), 123–29.

13. V. E. Uhley, M. A. Pellizzon, A. M. Buison, F. Guo, Z. Djuric, and K. L. Jen, "Chronic Weight Cycling Increases Oxidative DNA Damage Levels in Mammary Gland of Female Rats Fed a High-Fat Diet," *Nutrition and Cancer* 29, no. 1 (1997), 55–59. A. R. Tagliaferro, A. M. Ronan, L. D. Meeker, H. J. Thompson, A. L. Scott, "Cyclic Food Restriction, Insulin and Mammary Cell Proliferation in the Rat," *Carcinogenesis* 18, no. 11 (November 1997), 2271–76.

14. A. Settnes, T. Jorgensen, A. P. Lange, "Hysterectomy in Danish Women: Weight-Related Factors, Psychologic Factors, and Life-Style Variables," *Obstetrics and Gynecology* 88, no. 1 (July 1996), 99–105.

15. M. W. Green and P. J. Rogers, "Impaired Cognitive Functioning During Spontaneous Dieting," *Psychological Medicine* 25, no. 5 (September 1995), 1003–10.

16. S. H. Stewart, M. Angelopoulos, J. M. Baker, and F. J. Boland, "Relations Between Dietary Restraint and Patterns of Alcohol Use in Young Adult Women," *Psychology of Addictive Behavior* 14, no. 1 (March 2000), 77–82.

17. N. W. Brown, J. L. Treasure, and I. C. Campbell, "Evidence for Long-Term Pancreatic Damage Caused by Laxative Abuse in Subjects Recovered from Anorexia Nervosa," *International Journal of Eating Disorders* 29, no. 2 (March 2001), 236–38.

18. Carol Bloom and Laura Kogel, "Symbolic Meanings of Food and Body," *Eating Problems: A Feminist Psychoanalytic Treatment Model* (New York: BasicBooks, 1994), 58.

19. *Diagnostic and Statistical Manual of Mental Disorders*, Fourth Edition (Washington, D. C.: American Psychiatric Association, 2000).

20. K. A. Smith, C. G. Fairburn, and P. J. Cowen, "Symptomatic Relapse in Bulimia Nervosa Following Acute Tryptophan Depletion," *Archives of General Psychiatry* 56, no. 2 (February 1999), 171–76.

Chapter 3

1. Barbara Dafoe Whitehead, "The Girls of Gen X," *American Enterprise* (January/February 1998).

2. Silverstein, Peterson, Perdue, and Kelly, 1986, cited by Liz Dittrich in "About-Face Facts About the Media," @ about-face.org.

3. S. A. French, M. Story, G. Remafedi, M. D. Resnick, and R. W. Blum, "Sexual Orientation and Prevalence of Body Dissatisfaction and Eating Disordered Behaviors: A Population-Based Study of Adolescents," *International Journal of Eating Disorders* 19, no. 2 (March 1996), 119–26.

4. Study cited by Alicia Potter in "Mirror Image," *Weekly Wire* 1, no. 27 (December 1997).

5. Sandy Naiman, "Suck Out Your Gut," *Toronto Sun* (June 26, 1998).

6. Reported in a November 19, 1996 *New York Post* article cited on supermodel.com.

7. Study cited by Alicia Potter, in "Mirror Image," *Weekly Wire* 1, no. 27 (December 1997).

8. Susan Bordo, *Unbearable Weight: Feminism, Western Culture, and the Body* (Berkeley, CA: University of California Press, 1993), 57.

9. Liz Dittrich, "About-Face Facts on Body Image," @ about-face.org.

10. "NOW Foundation Says 'Love Your Body'" (1998). Press release.

11. Study cited by Susan Bordo in *Unbearable Weight*, 56.

12. Study cited by Susan Bordo in *Unbearable Weight*, 56.

13. Survey data are from Dale M. Atrens, *Don't Diet* (New York: William Morrow and Company, 1988), 109.

14. Kirsten Krahnstoever Davison and Leann Lipps Birch, "Weight Status, Parent Reaction, and Self-Concept in Five-Year-Old Girls," *Pediatrics* 107, no. 1 (January 2001), 46–53. Davison quoted by Elizabeth Mehren in "Body Image Weighs Heavily on Girls Even at Age 5, Study Says," *Los Angeles Times* (March 7, 2001).

15. Emily Bazelon, "She's Gotta Habit," *Education Week*, October 1997, @ edweek.org/tm/vol09/02smoke.h09.

16. C. A. Tomeo, A. E. Field, C. S. Berkey, G. A. Colditz, and A. L. Frazier. "Weight Concerns, Weight Control Behaviors, and Smoking Initiation," *Pediatrics* 104, no. 4 Pt. 1 (October 1999), 918–24.

17. Joyce Clark Hicks, "Crossing a Thin Line," *Raleigh News & Observer* (November 5, 1998).

18. Candace DePuy and Dana Dovitch, "Body Image," *Feminista!* 2, no. 6 (1998).

19. Tom Reynolds, "Sharp Rise in Disordered Eating in Fiji Follows Arrival of Western TV," *Harvard Focus* (May 28, 1999).

20. Study cited in Liz Dittrich, "About-Face Facts on SES, Ethnicity, and the Thin Ideal" (1997), @ about-face.org.

21. Douglas Yu and Glenn Shepard Jr. "Is Beauty in the Eye of the Beholder?" *Nature* 396 (November 1998), 321–22.

22. Susan Kano, *Making Peace with Food* (New York: Perennial Library, 1989), 39.

23. Statistic cited in Carol Bloom et al., eds., *Eating Problems: A Feminist Psychoanalytic Treatment Model* (New York: Basic Books, 1994), 72.

24. Bill Hoffmann, "The Skinny on Playboy Nudes: They're Too Thin," *New York Post* (December 13, 2000).

25. S. Rubinstein and B. Caballero, "Is Miss America an Undernourished Role Model?" *Journal of the American Medical Association* 283, no. 12 (March 22/29, 2000), 1569.

Chapter 4

1. Raena Morgan, "Diet Damage Control," *Her Health Online* (November 1998), @ herhealth.com/focus/bodyimage/dietdamage.html.

Chapter 5

1. "Most Young Women 'Unhappy with Bodies'," BBC News (February 21, 2001).
2. *Body Image and Advertising* (Studio City, CA: Mediascope Press, 2000). Issue Briefs.
3. D. M. Garner and S. C. Wolley, "Confronting the Failure of Behavioral and Dietary Treatments for Obesity," *Clinical Psychology Review* 11 (1991), 729–80.

Chapter 6

1. Erich Fromm, *The Art of Loving* (New York: Harper & Brothers, 1956), 54.
2. Carol Bloom and Laura Kogal, "Learning to Feed Ourselves," *Eating Problems: A Feminist Psychoanalytic Treatment Model* (New York: Basic Books, 1994), 114.
3. Erich Fromm, *The Art of Loving* (New York: Harper & Brothers, 1956), 116.
4. Erich Fromm, *The Art of Loving* (New York: Harper & Brothers, 1956), 5.

Chapter 7

1. Noreen Williams, "Let Hunger Be Your Diet Guide—and Your Daughter's," *Florida Today* 21, no. 32 (April 7, 1998).

Chapter 8

1. Joan Price, "Make Fitness Happen," @ joanprice.com.
2. Erich Fromm, *The Art of Loving* (New York: Harper & Brothers, 1956), 100–01.
3. Klaas R. Westerterp, "Pattern and Intensity of Physical Activity," *Nature* 410 (March 29, 2001), 539.

4. I-Min Lee, Kathryn Rexrode, Nancy Cook, JoAnne Manson, and Julie Buring, "Physical Activity and Coronary Heart Disease in Women: Is 'No Pain, No Gain' Passé?" *Journal of the American Medical Association* 285, no. 11 (March 21, 2001), 1447–54.

5. T. Hayashi, K. Tsumura, C. Suematsu, K. Okada, S. Fujii, and G. Endo, "Walking to Work and the Risk for Hypertension in Men: the Osaka Health Survey," *Annals of Internal Medicine* 131, no. 1 (July 6, 1999), 21–26.

6. Frank B. Hu, Ronald J. Sigal, Janet W. Rich-Edwards, Graham A. Colditz, Caren G. Solomon, Walter C. Willett, Frank E. Speizer, and JoAnne E. Manson, "Walking Compared with Vigorous Physical Activity and Risk of Type 2 Diabetes in Women," *Journal of the American Medical Association* 282 (October 20, 1999), 1433–39.

Chapter 9

1. Sydney Walker, *Dose of Sanity* (New York: Wiley & Sons, 1996).

Chapter 10

1. Judy A. McLean, Susan I. Barr, and Jerilynn C. Prior, "Cognitive Dietary Restraint Is Associated with Higher Urinary Cortisol Excretion in Healthy Premenopausal Women," *American Journal of Clinical Nutrition* 73, no. 1 (January 2001), 7–12.

2. E. Epel, R. Lapidus, B. McEwen, and K. Brownell, "Stress May Add Bite to Appetite in Women: A Laboratory Study of Stress-Induced Cortisol and Eating Behavior," *Psychoneuroendocrinology* 26, no. 1 (January 2001), 37–49.

3. G. S. Birketvedt, J. Florholmen, J. Sundsfjord, B. Osterud, D. Dinges, W. Bilker, and A. Stunkard, "Behavioral and Neuroendorine Characteristics of the Night-Eating Syndrome," *Journal of the American Medical Association* 282 (August 18, 1999), 657–63.

4. E. Doucet, P. Imbeault, S. St. Pierre, N. Almeras, P. Mauriege, D. Richard, and A. Tremblay, "Appetite After Weight Loss by Energy Restriction and a Low-Fat Diet-Exercise Follow-Up," *International Journal of Obesity and Related Metabolic Disorders* 24, no. 7 (July 2000), 906–14.

5. Erich Fromm, *The Art of Loving* (New York: Harper & Brothers, 1956), 99.

Chapter 11

1. "Di's Private Battle: The Princess's Struggle with Bulimia Brings a Puzzling Disease out of the Shadows," *Time* (August 3, 1992).
2. Peg McNulty, "Eating Disorders Among a Population of Navy Men Who? When? Why?" updated research for Navy Nurse corps, @ nmcsd.med.navy.mil/support/nursingresearch/mnult4.html.

Chapter 12

1. Thorne-Smith's comments to *U.S. Weekly* cited by Michael Ausiello in "The Skinny on Courtney Thorne-Smith," *TV Guide*, December 5, 2000.
2. Naomi Wolf, "Dying to Be Thin: The Prevention of Eating Disorders and the Role of Federal Policy." Address to the United States Congress, July 1997.

Chapter 13

1. Booker T. Washington, *The Story of My Life and Work* (Naperville, IL: Nichols and Company, c1900).
2. From "The Doctor's Office," All Children's Hospital website, @ allkids.org/Epstein/Articles/Obese_Children.html.
3. Doug Brunk, "Type 2 Diabetes Is Growing Problem in Children and Teens," *Pediatric News* 33, no. 9 (1999), 1.
4. American Diabetes Association, "Why Are Children Being Diagnosed with a 'Middle Aged' Disease?" *Diabetes Forecast* (December 1998), @ diabetes.org/DiabetesForecast/98Dec/pg46.asp.
5. Amy Dickinson, "Measuring Up," *Time* 156, no. 21 (November 20, 2000).
6. Martha Irvine, "Weight Fears Growing for Younger Girls," *Chicago Sun-Times* (July 23, 2001).
7. Michael Loewy, "Working with Fat Children in Schools," *Radiance Online* (Fall 1998), @ radiancemagazine.com.

8. Paul Kendall, "How Does Your Dieting Influence Your Child?" *Daily Mail* (September 2000). Research reported by John Reilly et al. at the "Update on Childhood Nutrition" conference, September 6, 2000, University of Glasgow, Scotland.

9. J. O. Fisher and L. L. Birch, "Restricting Access to Palatable Foods Affects Children's Behavioral Response, Food Selection, and Intake," *American Journal of Clinical Nutrition* 69, no. 6 (June 1999), 1264–72.

10. Findings reported by Leann Birch at the Update on Childhood Nutrition Conference, September 6, 2000, University of Glasgow, Scotland.

11. R. E. Kreipe and G. B. Forbes, "Osteoporosis: A 'New Morbidity' for Dieting Female Adolescents?" *Pediatrics* 86, no. 3 (September 1990), 478–80.

12. "Researcher Warns Diets for Overweight Children May Stunt Growth," *Doctor's Guide* (April 13, 1998), @ pslgroup.com.

13. G. C. Patton, J. B. Carlin, Q. Shao, M. E. Hibbert, M. Rosier, R. Selzer, and G. Bowes, "Adolescent Dieting: Healthy Weight Control or Borderline Eating Disorder?" *Journal of Child Psychology and Psychiatry* 38, no. 3 (March 1997), 299–306. K. A. Bruinsma and D. L. Taren, "Dieting, Essential Fatty Acid Intake, and Depression," *Nutrition Review* 58, no. 4 (April 2000), 98–108.

14. Ann B. Bruner, Alain Joffee, Anne K. Duggan, F. Casella, and Jason Brandt. "Randomised Study of Cognitive Effects of Iron Supplementation in Non-Anaemic Iron-Deficient Adolescent Girls," *The Lancet* 347, no. 9033 (October 12, 1996), 992–6. M. W. Green and P. J. Rogers, "Impaired Cognitive Functioning During Spontaneous Dieting," *Psychological Medicine* 25, no. 5 (September 1995), 1003–10.

15. G. C. Patton, R. Selzer, C. Coffey, J. B. Carlin, and R. Wolfe, "Onset of Adolescent Eating Disorders: Population Based Cohort Study over 3 Years," *British Medical Journal* 318 (March 20, 1999), 765–68.

16. B. Lowe, S. Zipfel, C. Buchholz, Y. Dupont, D. L. Reas, and W. Herzog, "Long-Term Outcome of Anorexia Nervosa in a Prospective 21-Year Follow-Up Study," *Psychological Medicine* 31, no. 5 (July 2001), 881–90.

17. S. L. Gortmaker, A. Must, A. M. Sobol, K. Peterson, G. A. Colditz, and W. H. Dietz, "Television Viewing as a Cause of Increasing Obesity Among Children in the United States, 1986–1990," *Archives of Pediatric and Adolescent Medicine* 150, no. 4 (April 1996), 356–62.

INDEX

227

ABOUT THE AUTHOR

WENDY OLIVER-PYATT is a practicing psychiatrist and assistant professor at the University of Nevada-Reno. She completed her psychiatry training at New York University, where she was chief resident of the Bellvue Hospital Outpatient Service. Dr. Oliver-Pyatt has held faculty positions at NYU, Albert Einstein School of Medicine, and the University of Nevada School of Medicine. She has taught courses on food and body preoccupation to medical students, psychiatry residents, and other health-care providers. Board certified by the American Board of Psychiatry and Neurology in both general and addiction psychiatry, Dr. Oliver-Pyatt has appeared on television programs as an expert on dieting, eating disorders, and related topics. She is a frequent lecturer and currently resides in Reno, Nevada, with her husband and two daughters.